Turning the World Upside Down: the search for global health in the twenty-first century

Nigel Crisp

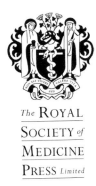

The ROYAL
SOCIETY of
MEDICINE
PRESS Limited

Published by the Royal Society of Medicine Press Ltd
1 Wimpole Street, London W1G 0AE, UK
Tel: +44 (0)20 7290 2921
Fax: +44 (0)20 7290 2929
E-mail: publishing@rsmpress.ac.uk
Website: www.rsmpress.co.uk

British Library Cataloguing in Publication Data
A catalogue record for this book is available from the British Library

ISBN: 978-1-85315-933-6

Distribution in Europe and Rest of the World:
Marston Book Services Ltd
PO Box 269
Abingdon
Oxon OX14 4YN, UK
Tel: +44 (0)1235 465500
Fax: +44 (0)1235 465555
Email: direct.order@marston.co.uk

Distribution in USA and Canada:
Royal Society of Medicine Press Ltd
c/o BookMasters Inc
30 Amberwood Parkway
Ashland, OH 44805, USA
Tel: +1 800 247 6553/ +1 800 266 5564
Fax: +1 410 281 6883
Email: order@bookmasters.com

Distribution in Australia and New Zealand:
Elsevier Australia
30–52 Smidmore Street
Marrickville NSW 2204, Australia
Tel: +61 2 9517 8999
Fax: +61 2 9517 2249
Email: service@elsevier.com.au

Phototypeset by MTC Manila
Cover photograph by Kate Holt reproduced by permission of Sightsavers International
Some figures by Jonathan Bosley of HLM Architects
Project Management by Aileen Castell of Naughton Project Management
Printed in India by Replika Press Pvt. Ltd.

Contents

Preface

There are two simple ideas at the very heart of this book – that rich countries can learn a great deal about health and health services from poorer ones and that combining the learning from rich and poor countries can give us new insight into how to improve health.

Having run the world's biggest health service, England's NHS, for more than 5 years, I was asked by Prime Minister Blair to look at how we could use all the accumulated experience and expertise about health which we had in the UK to improve health in developing countries. As I travelled the world at his request, meeting people and visiting services, I began to see that there were indeed many ways in which we could help, that many British health workers and organisations wanted to help and, indeed, many were already doing so.

I also began to realise, however, that creative, passionate local people in countries that didn't have our resources, were innovating, finding solutions and working out how to use the materials at hand to provide the best deal they could for their patients. Unconstrained by our history, conventions and institutions, they were training people differently, creating new types of organisations, involving families and communities, and concentrating much more on promoting health and independence rather than on just tackling disease.

There is no comparison, of course, between the problems to be found in the poorest parts of the world and those in rich countries like the UK. Ill health, poverty, life expectancy and disability are all so much worse in the poorer countries. People die and are damaged by some of the simplest and most treatable or preventable diseases and situations. It is plain to see that science, technology, medicine, professionalism, knowledge and systems, combined with more resources and health workers are desperately needed. It is also plain and obvious, however, that health systems in rich countries are in trouble. Whilst poorer countries need more of what we in richer countries have – our science and expertise – perhaps we also need more of what they have learned.

This very simple idea has led me to recognise that talking about developing and developed countries and about international development can be very misleading. We all have something to learn and all have something to teach. We are in this together and we will develop together. I have used instead the expressions richer and poorer countries and, in doing so, recognised that there is a spectrum. There are very rich and very poor and many in between, all of them with their own particular circumstances and features – however it is the richer that have most of the power and who determine the way the world's institutions and relationships work, and the poorer who have to live within a world shaped by others.

I have used many examples and illustrations from my own experience and observations – drawing on my time in the NHS and my experiences working on global programmes to train more health workers in poorer countries. I have also used examples from my role as Chair of Sightsavers International, which works with local partners in 33 countries to prevent blindness, treat eye disease and help blind and partially sighted people live as independent lives as possible.

I am grateful to the many people who have allowed me to tell a part of their story and to them and the many others from whom I have learned. I have used their examples to bring the book to life and ground it in reality.

Turning the World Upside Down is in many ways a description of what is happening now and of the things which innovative health workers, leaders and politicians are doing today. It describes people learning how to work more effectively and how to have a greater impact and is written in conscious admiration of the many millions of health workers worldwide who work with such compassion, determination and imagination. They, not I, are the people who are creating the new vision for health that I describe in this book.

I am deeply grateful to many people who have taught me about their countries and continents including Francis Omaswa, Bience Gawanas, Fazle Hassan Abed and Srinath Reddy as well as to Don Berwick, Maureen Bisognano and colleagues from the Institute for Healthcare Improvement for their inspiration and insight; Mary Robinson, Peggy Clark and colleagues from Realizing Rights for helping me understand human rights and health; Michael Birt and colleagues at the Pacific Health Summit for introducing me to new ideas; Margaret Chan, Tim Evans and colleagues at the World Health Organization; Joy Phumaphi, Julian Schweitzer and colleagues from the World Bank; and Ernest Massiah, Peggy Vidot and colleagues from the Commonwealth Secretariat, for their continuing support and guidance.

I have been privileged to work with many people in The Global Health Workforce Alliance and the Gates Foundation and to have been accompanied on my earlier travels by Imogen Sharp and Amy Kesterton. Throughout, I have also been very fortunate to have been able to call on help from so many people in the UK's Department for International Development and Foreign Office; both of whom have proved to be unparalleled sources of insight and understanding. It has been a pleasure to see how highly they are regarded in the countries where they work. The UK is a global leader in international development. I am also very fortunate to have been able to call on help from the Department of Health and benefit from the expertise of many of its staff.

I am also indebted to the people who read and improved parts of this book who include, as well as some of the above, John Bacon, Kate Barnard, Vivian Bazalgette, Ali Enayati, Ruth English, Phil Freeman, David Jenkins, Anna Maslin, Joe McCannon, Debbie Mellor, Eldryd Parry, David Percy and Paddy Salmon.

Susana Edjang has done an outstanding job as my researcher, providing me with the evidence, analysis and references I needed and offering me her own insight. The book is much the richer for her contribution.

Finally and above all, I am grateful to Siân, Madeleine and Alastair for their advice on science and anthropology and their – almost – unqualified understanding and support over the last year.

Nigel Crisp

Tutts Clump
December 2009

List of Abbreviations Used

ACE	Angiotensin-converting enzyme
AIDS	Acquired immune deficiency syndrome
ANC	African National Congress
API	Associates in Performance Improvement
ART	Anti-Retroviral Therapy
ASHAs	Accredited Social Health Workers
BRAC	Bangladesh Rural Action Committee
CAN	Community Action Network
DFID	Department for International Development
DVT	Deep vein thrombosis
FDA	Food and Drug Administration
GAVI	Global Action on Vaccination and Immunization
GSK	GlaxoSmithKline
HIPC	Highly Indebted Poor Countries Initiative
HIV	Human immunodeficiency virus
ICT	information and communication technology
IFMSA	International Federation of Medical Student Associations
IHI	Institute for Healthcare Improvement
IHP	International Health Partnerships
IMF	International Monetary Fund
MCN	Movimiento Comunal Nicaragüense
MDRI	Multilateral Debt Relief Initiative
MHRA	Medicines and Healthcare products Regulatory Agency
MMR	Measles, mumps and rubella
MOH	Ministry of Health
MRSA	Methicillin-resistant *Staphylococcus aureus*
NGO	Non-governmental organisation
NICE	National Institute for Health and Clinical Excellence
PAHO	Pan American Organization for Health
PEPFAR	President's Emergency Plan for AIDS Relief
SARS	Severe Acute Respiratory Syndrome
SCF	South Central Foundation
TB	Tuberculosis
THET	Tropical Health Education Trust
UN	United Nations
URC	University Research Company
USAID	United States Agency for International Development
WHO	World Health Organization

1 Introduction

Diseases travel; the microbe that boards a plane in Cambodia this morning can be in Washington before the sun has set. The Internet provides information and knowledge but also spreads ignorance, prejudice and superstition to every part of the world. Science and technology create enormous benefit but can also bring new environmental and biological perils, which, like climate change, will affect us all.

The most striking thing about health in the twenty-first century is that the whole world is now so interconnected and so interdependent. This interdependence is changing the way we see health, creating a new global perspective and will affect the way we need to act.

Turning the World Upside Down is a search to understand what is happening and what it means for us. It is based on my own journey from running the largest health system in the world to working in some of the poorest countries and draws on my experience and experiences to explore new ideas and innovations from around the world.

It argues that western scientific medicine, which has been such a dominant and successful force in the world, is no longer by itself capable of continuing to improve our health. We need to understand how to make the best use of our ever-improving scientific knowledge and technology. Unless we take account of the new global dimension we will be in constant danger of using twentieth-century ideas and tools to tackle twenty-first-century problems. We need a paradigm shift towards a global perspective, towards global health.

This chapter sets the scene, describes the wider context and discusses global health itself, by which we mean everything that affects us all, wherever we live, from global warming and the spread of disease to the migration of health workers and the availability of medicines.

The search for understanding

Our search for understanding starts by looking at the current state of health and healthcare in the different parts of the world. A simple story illustrates just how successful western scientific medicine has been and how much health has improved for the populations of rich western countries in the last century.

Life in the mountains and valleys of South Wales was much tougher in the 1920s and 1930s than it is today and life expectancy was shorter. Half the population didn't reach retirement age, about 1 in 250 women died in childbirth, there was no health system for the poor and tuberculosis (TB) was rampant. It must have seemed to many people that things would never improve.

Ben Jenkins owned and operated a timber yard in Brecon and lived next door to it with his wife, nine children and a maid. They were a relatively prosperous family and lived a very different life from the miners in the valleys nearby, who were constantly at risk from work-related diseases and the dangers of the coal mines. They were not poor and could afford to call the doctor; nevertheless, the Jenkins family faced tragedy.

Trevor, the eldest child, caught TB whilst working away from home and died aged 21 in 1929. Tragically, he had brought the disease home with him and most of the family were affected. Several were sent to sanatoria higher in the mountains and two went to Switzerland in an effort to recover or escape the disease altogether. The treatment was only partially successful and Ben and both his daughters, Winifred and Betty, died of TB in the following years.

David, the seventh son and youngest child recalls being sent to a sanatorium for a whole year at the age of 8 in 1931. His mother, who by this time had seen her husband and others of her children sicken, couldn't bear to say goodbye to another one, possibly for the last time, so the small boy found himself sent away with strangers in a vast hospital not knowing what was happening to him and unable to communicate with his family.

The other children lived but the mother died, of a broken heart according to family legend, although in reality of a brain tumour, in the week that her youngest child, David, went off to join his remaining brothers at war in 1942.

It was not just TB that was such a killer at the time. The story in those Welsh hills was that one funeral led to another. Standing hatless in the rain mourners were at risk of pneumonia, still a regular killer in those pre-antibiotic days.

Today, having survived the risks of TB, pneumonia and war, my father-in-law David Jenkins is 85. Three of his elder brothers, two in their 90s, attended his and Elaine's 60th wedding anniversary party last year. The Jenkins family can trace the story of how health has been transformed in the UK through the history of their own family, where the eldest died young and the youngest survive today.

The experience of the Jenkins family was by no means unique and life expectancy in the UK increased by 30 years in the last century. That is 3 years in every decade or almost 8 hours more for every day that we lived. One need only translate this through into one's own life to see how significant this is. My life expectancy at birth was about 65. It is now above 80. I am truly very grateful to all concerned.

It's not just about life expectancy, of course. We are healthier and fitter in our 50s, 60s, 70s and 80s and beyond than our parents were at the same age. We have 'wonder' drugs that allow us to manage our heart disease and other conditions and we have replacement hips, knees and lenses that give us so much more freedom from our disabilities. We are much richer now as a society in the UK and therefore much more able to acquire labour-saving, life-enhancing devices and drugs than at any time in human history.

We can see how health has improved enormously over the last century but we can also see that continuing growth in health services and funding is now only producing marginal benefits. It is the same story in many rich countries where massive increases in expenditure in recent years, planned as in the UK or unplanned as in the USA, have led to improvements but have not transformed health services. At the same time the public is becoming more assertive, harder to please and less willing simply to follow medical advice and be passive and patient.

Looking more deeply we can see that part of the reason for these problems and the dissatisfaction of the public is that the most significant diseases of the twenty-first century in richer countries are different from those in the twentieth century so that our health services have to deal with different problems.

We are no longer generally so affected by the communicable diseases like TB; infections are better controlled, there is less injury and accidental death and many cancers are becoming manageable chronic diseases. It is now these long-term conditions and noncommunicable diseases, such as cancers, heart disease and diabetes that require the most attention and use the most resources.

There need to be new and very different ways of dealing with these diseases – with more services created outside hospital, more involvement of the patient and much greater integration into other aspects of the patient's life such as education, employment and leisure activities. Many, perhaps most, clinicians and health workers have tried to change their practice accordingly. However, as I can describe from my own experience in the NHS, it is very difficult in practice to change the way healthcare is delivered.

A major part of the difficulty is that the very factors that led to such improvements in the twentieth century – the essential features of western scientific medicine: scientific discovery, greater professionalism, commercial innovation and massively increased funding – are so invested in maintaining and developing the old models of delivery and behaviour that they make it difficult to create new ones and are themselves becoming part of the problem.

We have built up over the years such tremendously strong health systems that they condition what we can do in practice and, in effect, dictate what happens when people are ill. As a result we may end up in hospital when we don't need to. We may be overinvestigated, overmedicated and, in all likelihood, overspent.

More problematically these features of western scientific medicine have also conditioned our mindsets so that we have a very simple model in our minds of what good treatment looks like. We have come to expect treatment by doctors with the latest equipment and drugs in specialist facilities and hospitals, whether or not this is actually what we need for our particular problem or illness. Good treatment for our condition may actually be something else altogether.

The dominance of this way of thinking amongst politicians, health leaders and the public is so great that most attempts at reforming health systems in richer countries have concentrated on getting the best out of the existing model, through improving the existing arrangements, incentivising doctors differently and making more productive use of equipment and facilities. These reforms have not, despite great rhetoric, generally led in any major way to designing completely different services and systems suitable for the longer term conditions and chronic diseases we now face, let alone produced a major swing towards health promotion and disease prevention.

Existing power structures and vested interests reinforce this dominance at every turn. Almost any change, any innovation and any improvement will disadvantage somebody. Moving services to the community reduces hospital income. The empowerment of nurses and patients, which may be necessary to improve health, reduces the power of the doctors and commercial companies.

Whilst many doctors, hospital chief executives and businesses, as I shall describe in later chapters, are leading innovators and driving many of the improvements in the world, their professional and business associations recognise the threat to their power bases and react accordingly by opposing the change. This has happened time and again over the years, as when the UK's British Medical Association, the doctors' trade union, opposed the establishment of the NHS in 1948 until they were bought off, their "mouths stuffed with gold" in the words of the NHS founder Aneurin Bevin.

This history shows that it requires not only great political leadership and resolve to drive change in a complex field like health but also consummate political skill to generate support and energy and negotiate around the obstacles. Politicians around the world know to their cost just how difficult this can be.

From Wales to Bangladesh

Turning to low- and middle-income countries we find that in many of them, just like in Wales in the 1920s, half the population does not reach the equivalent of retirement age, 1 in 250 women die in childbirth, there is no health system for the poor and TB is rampant. It must seem to many people that things will never improve.

I recalled the Jenkins family history as I flew back from Bangladesh in 2008 and thought about the poverty and the illness I had seen there. What were the chances of a similar transformation in Bangladesh, I wondered? More importantly, why wasn't it already happening? We know what to do clinically about all the most common diseases and problems. There has been an enormous investment in aid and development. It seemed outrageous that it wasn't just happening. What was getting in the way?

I had begun to think about these issues when the Prime Minister, Tony Blair, had asked me to consider what more the UK could do to use its experience and expertise to help improve health in developing countries.[1] I had reported to him in 2007 but had remained involved in health globally. On this occasion, as Chair of Sightsavers, I had been visiting eye services in Bangladesh and had been reminded by my visit of the enormous contrast there was between health in richer and poorer countries.

I had spent more than 5 years as the Chief Executive of England's National Health Service. It is the largest integrated health service and the fourth biggest organisation in the world with 1.3 million employees and a turnover of almost £100 billion a year. Only the Chinese Army, the Indian railways and Wal-Mart are larger.

In some ways these organisations seem to reflect the countries themselves. They draw attention to China's power, India's size and the restless movement of its populations, and America's love of commerce. For the UK, the NHS undoubtedly represents something about us as a nation. It is a universal system; mainly tax funded, which is designed to offer services to every citizen, equally, regardless of their ability to pay. Love it or hate it, the NHS says something about the British and our ideas about fairness and compassion.

On that flight from Bangladesh I was coming home from a country that has a very different way of life and a very different health system, where the majority of the services provided for the poor aren't run or sponsored by the Government but by the Bangladesh

Rural Action Committee (BRAC). BRAC is a voluntary organisation, possibly the largest non-governmental organisation (NGO) in the world, which brings together literally millions of Bangladeshis in local groups to plan and organise services.

BRAC doesn't just deal with health, but with education and other public services as well. It runs empowerment groups for women, teaching them how to take action to better their lives and those of their families. It has its own microfinance bank to provide small loans to enable people, mainly women, to earn a living, allowing them to purchase seed or farming tools or to buy goods that they can sell on in the local markets. It runs a university and shops and is prepared to be involved and invest in any practical approaches that benefit the poor.

BRAC is a remarkable example of people who are not prepared to wait for others to help them but have taken the future into their own hands and are creating their own solutions. The way they do things challenges the top-down, professionalised and commercialised mindset that is so common in richer countries. Even this short description shows just how differently services are organized in Bangladesh from the model described earlier.

Funding is also managed differently. In Bangladesh, as in several other low-income countries, I saw microfinance systems paying out loans for healthcare and a system of cross-subsidy in place where those who were able to were expected to pay for their services, whilst the poorest got them free. Everyone, however, received the same attention and the same clinical service.

BRAC, like the NHS, represents an idea, an ideal and a sense of justice and community. It was founded in 1972 during the country's struggles for independence from Pakistan and embodies the values of self-determination and self-sufficiency of that period. At the very same time that we had been agonising in the NHS over issues like the proper use of new and expensive technology and of how to get the best value from major new expenditure, BRAC was struggling in Bangladesh with the consequences of poverty and neglect and the problem of providing the most basic healthcare to a large part of their population.

Self-determination and self-help, so well exemplified by BRAC and other organisations, is a major theme of *Turning the World Upside Down* and will be referred to in later chapters. For the moment, however, let us return to my own question of why, despite the efforts of inspiring organisations like BRAC and despite the years of aid, big improvements were not already happening? Three reasons stand out. There are three levels of problems to confront at the same time; each is formidable and together they show how extremely difficult it is to make a truly transformational change.

Firstly, dealing purely with health issues, there is simply very much more disease and very many more causes of disease, injury and death than we now see in richer countries. Communicable diseases such as malaria, TB and human immunodeficiency virus (HIV)/acquired immune deficiency syndrome (AIDS) are rife in many countries, the non-communicable diseases are becoming more common and injury and death from conflict, traffic accidents and employment are widespread. Sub-Saharan Africa alone, with one tenth of the world's population has almost one-quarter of the world's burden of diseases.

At the second level, poverty affects health in myriad ways and makes it much harder to make improvements. One billion people around the world live in desperate poverty on less than a dollar a day; another billion scrape a living with little more than two dollars a day. It is not, of course, as if the dollar or two are available every day: some days it may be more, some days less or nothing. They are living on the edge and can easily be pushed over it into destitution, famine and death by disease, climate or war.

The health of many of the poorest people in the poorest countries is truly dreadful. The statistics are now so often repeated that they can easily be ignored; unless, of course, you decide to make it personal by thinking about your own children or relatives when you hear that one in five children die before the age of 5 in some parts of Sub-Saharan Africa.[2] It is almost worse to know that most of these deaths could so easily be avoided, even in the poorest countries, if there were clean water, insecticide-treated mosquito bed nets, adequate food and housing and better access to simple treatment, advice and education. All of these contribute to health whilst their absence leaves the way clear for illness, disability and death. People need more than just health services to improve their health.

Poverty also means that in many countries there is no health system to speak of, with few facilities and with difficulties in staffing and providing drugs, particularly in rural areas. Where health systems in richer countries may be too strong, they are often perilously weak in poorer ones and access to care may be haphazard, of uncertain quality and, where available, very costly.

At the third and deepest level we can also see how social, economic and political factors affect health profoundly within a country. The education of women is crucial in securing the health of their children whilst their own position in society often dictates whether they can – or are allowed to by their men folk – get access to trained health workers or whether they must instead use traditional healers and remedies. This contributes to the fact that over half a million women each year die in low- and middle-income countries in childbirth or as a result of pregnancy.[3]

Maternal death is the very epitome of a twenty-first-century problem. It is about social and economic factors as much as it is about the availability of appropriate treatment and healthcare. Indeed, given that the clinical care and treatment of pregnant women is so well understood, the social factors are the most significant and intractable barrier to improvement. It is a statement of the obvious, real 'motherhood and apple pie', that mothers are crucial to good health. They protect the health of their families. They educate and train their children in healthy habits. They lead health improvement efforts in any community. Their death or absence almost always means the absence of emotional security and stability and has long-term detrimental effects on their children.

Internationally we can see that there is a similar pattern whereby social, economic and political factors tend to make it harder for poorer countries to grow and develop. The most obvious example is the way economic and trade relationships are concentrated among the wealthiest regions of the world. They keep the money flowing and growing largely amongst themselves to the exclusion of poorer countries. In 2006, Europe, North America and Asia accounted for 86% and 90% of the world's merchandise exports and imports and 91% and 89% of the world's commercial services exports and imports.[4]

Africa's share, a region that comprises 53 countries, was only 3% of the world manufacturing exports and 2% of the world's commercial services.[4] Moreover, the bigger economies are also better able to subsidise their own producers at the expense of others. To take one simple example, the USA subsidised its own agricultural producers by US$31.6

billion in 2007 and as a result drove down international prices in commodities such as cotton to the disadvantage of many much poorer countries. Such subsidies far outweigh the USA's total overseas development aid, which amounted to US$25.8 billion in 2008, net of bilateral debt relief.[5]

In addition, poor countries have little access to capital, are worse affected by trade fluctuations and don't have the power and the positions in world organisations to lobby and negotiate effectively.[6] Their citizens generally have the poorer and less well-paid jobs in international organisations and processes. They are disproportionately the miners not the manufacturers, the farmers not the processors and, in the worst cases, the exploited child and adult labour not the protected workforce.

In health itself, as we shall see later, there is a particularly unfair import–export business where rich countries import trained health workers from poor countries and export their ideas and ideologies about healthcare to them in return. It is not a fair trade. Trained workers from poor countries emigrate to find their fortunes, leaving their homeland the poorer for the loss of the investment in their training as well as their talent. Richer countries, in turn, export their ideas and ideologies about health and medicine alongside their aid. In many cases, these ideas and ideologies are inappropriate and may be out of date and discredited in their countries of origin.

It is not just in health, of course, that ideas and ideologies are exported with aid and development. The major donors and development agencies have moved beyond the idea of simple charity and doing things to and for people towards the idea of helping them to do things for themselves. In practice, however, this is still very often a purely one-way relationship with donors and development agencies deciding what happens in a country, sometimes regardless of the wishes of the country itself. There is still little idea of accountability to the recipient country and virtually no conception of mutual benefit.

International aid and development is itself going through a period of great change at the moment. The established agencies and donors, largely from western democracies, have created one pattern of giving that, in theory at least, is consistent across the world. Even they, however, have had their differences, with the USA, until the recent change of administration, standing apart from the liberal consensus of donor countries because of its refusal to promote condoms and abortion as means of population control.

The other great and emerging powers of China, India, Russia and to some extent, Brazil, have different ideas and are engaging in bilateral negotiations with poorer countries to gain preferential trade agreements and secure natural resources. Oil and minerals are great attractions for investors, but so, too, are land and the food it can produce. Sudan, Ethiopia, Congo and Pakistan are among the countries that have leased over 20 million hectares of farmland, an area almost half the size of Spain, to foreigners who use it to grow food for their own populations and not for the locals, however hungry.[7]

Global health

This discussion of the relationships involved in international development leads naturally to a discussion of what we mean by global health. Here, I am taking it to embrace all those health issues that affect us all, rich and poor.

There are many such issues, with the most obvious being that we share a vulnerability to epidemics of diseases that can affect our economy and international relationships as well as our health. We need only remember how Severe Acute Respiratory Syndrome (SARS) incubated in the Guangdong province in rural China in November 2002. By June 2003 it had killed 33 people in Toronto, Canada, 12 000 miles away and was damaging world trade.

As I write in the summer of 2009, the first wave of H1N1 or 'swine flu', originating in Mexico, has swept around the world, bringing with it sickness and terror. The Black Death took about three years to travel across Europe in the mid 1300s; swine flu took about 3 days to circle the world and to set every health ministry and international organisation into a whirl of activity and every government into emergency sessions on whether to close their airports and borders and quarantine travellers. It is too early to know what impact the second and further waves will have although we can be sure that contingency plans to deal with them are being developed around the world.

I well remember sitting in the Department of Health's 'War Room' in London's Whitehall as we role-played our responses to outbreaks of global disease. We concentrated for part of the time on the disease itself and how, with our international partners, to identify and treat it and develop new vaccines and treatments. We spent as much time, however, on managing its wider impacts: thinking about how to inform the public, what to do if France or other neighbours closed their borders and what advice to give hospital, schools and employers. It went far beyond the normal confines of a discussion on health.

SARS and H1N1 are real-life examples, but it does not take much imagination to recognise the potential of other threats. There will be other 'zoonotic' diseases created through the interaction of animal and human viruses. One of these, one day, may well prove just too powerful and too infectious for it to be contained by all our efforts and as a result kill millions around the world. We can also easily imagine how terrorists or, indeed, rogue governments and armies could use biological agents to blackmail, disable and kill.

Health security, our ability to reduce and manage these natural and man-made threats, has become a matter of concern to us all. We are now beginning to understand fully that the health of one nation affects its neighbours and that we need to share our knowledge and build our defences together. We are only as strong as our weakest part, wherever that may be.

Lincoln Chen and Vasant Narasimhan of Harvard University draw attention to this in a wide-ranging submission for the Commission on Human Security in 2002. They point out that under the very visible health threats that we can all easily understand will affect us all – such as disease outbreaks and bio-terrorism – there are much larger hidden epidemics of more common diseases and health failures which already exist and that affect the poor. If these are not tackled, they can breed personal and national insecurity and, of course, incubate new strains and diseases. They illustrate this with the analogy of an iceberg: part is visible; a larger part is hidden (Figure 1.1).[8]

We see this very clearly in the way that a new strain of multidrug-resistant TB is spreading rapidly around the globe. This, a variant of the disease that killed the older Jenkins siblings in Wales in the 1920s, is no longer treatable with our ordinary antibiotics but requires the development of new generations of drugs. TB, which was once beaten in most of the world, will have to be beaten again. It had become a disease of the poor, forgotten and invisible to the rest of the world in the 'submerged' part of the iceberg described by

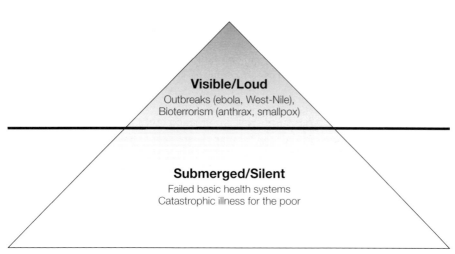

Figure 1.1 The iceberg analogy. From Chen and Narasimhan 2002

Chen and Narasimhan. Now it is a real threat to us all and, 'visible' one again, requires massive effort to limit its reach and reduce its potentially devastating impact.[9]

The impact of climate change is potentially even greater than any of these other problems. It is likely to affect many of the poorer countries first, with Africa suffering the loss of fertile country and water and parts of Bangladesh potentially disappearing beneath the sea. There may be some short term benefits in some parts of the world. However, the subsequent impact of reduced food yields, reduced biodiversity, less drinkable water, the movement of populations, conflict over resources and higher sea levels is likely to affect us all. The continuing growth in population and its distribution around the world, a problem in itself, can only make matters worse.

Climate change has now become one of the biggest issues in global health with leading figures describing it variously as a potential global health catastrophe and the cholera of our era.[10–12] It is a shared problem that requires shared action.

The wider concept and concerns of global health

The concept of global health goes far wider than merely our shared vulnerability, important as this is. It embraces everything that we share in health terms globally. We are becoming more interdependent in terms of regulation with many international bodies attempting to set standards for everything from disease prevention to professional practice and the sharing of medical records. There is an international convention on the control of tobacco, standard definitions of health professions adhered to in much of the world, and an overwhelming amount of advice available on how to deliver services from authorities of all sorts.

We are interdependent, too, in terms of key health resources. We are dependent on the same relatively few pharmaceutical companies for certain drugs and the development of vaccines and, equally crucially, on the same pool of trained health workers, who may migrate from country to country. There is growing pressure internationally to share both these drugs and these health workers more equitably between the populations of the world.

Most profoundly of all, perhaps, we are connected together through shared knowledge about health, shared assumptions and shared behaviours. Western scientific medicine has become over the last century the dominant world model, moulding minds, habits and institutions in its image. It has largely rolled over and ignored other traditions, whether they are Islamic, Chinese or local, and become the model of choice on every continent. The environment is now changing, however, with a resurgence of interest in other ideas and the recognition that western scientific medicine cannot by itself solve every problem and deal with every situation.

Looking further afield, global health is also affected by the much wider considerations of economics and international relationships. Like swine flu the credit crunch swept around the world very rapidly, after a long incubation in the excesses of the 1990s and early 2000s. We are very far from knowing what the effects of the credit crunch will be on health and health care, even in the midterm. However, we can make some educated guesses that fear and turmoil will breed distress and ill health and that the growth in health expenditure in both rich and poor countries will be slowed. We can already see some of the impact on poorer countries with Italy and France cutting international development and the UK's contribution reduced sharply because the devaluation of sterling means each pound can buy less.

We don't yet know, either, how foreign policy and international relations will develop; beyond recognizing that power is shifting from west to east and that the policies of the big new economies of China, India, Russia and Brazil will have greater international significance and impact.

Recent commentators have variously suggested that it is by no means certain that any new power is yet ready to step into the space left by the West as it fades; that China's own internal conflicts will weaken its global dominance; that there will be a struggle for dominance between China, Japan and India; and that the USA's geo-political position, with coasts and ports on two oceans, will keep it dominant for longer than many now think.[13–15] Moreover, Russia and Brazil should not be forgotten.

The only thing that is clear is that there will be change. Perhaps the most telling point is made by Martin Jacques, the leading political commentator when he says: "the Chinese do not think of themselves as a nation but a civilization". The changes we can expect are not just about economics and power but will be about how power is exercised and about ideas and culture and behaviour. It won't just be a straight swap of superpowers; the rules of the game will change.

The credit crunch and these uncertainties have stimulated questions about the future role of the great international institutions such as the UN and its constituent bodies, like the World Health Organization, and the 'Bretton Woods' institutions such as the World Bank and the International Monetary Fund. These were all designed in the wake of twentieth-century crises in order to bring peace, economic and financial security and sustained development to the world. There is a need for re-design, this time with some of the emerging powers playing a bigger role in the new configuration and the way they work.

We have also witnessed the extraordinary spectacle in the UK, the USA and some other richer countries of the nationalisation or part nationalisation of banks. We appear to be seeing a changing of the balance between state and enterprise with the state playing a stronger role in the relationship in a way more familiar in eastern and emerging economies.

All of this adds to the continuing change brought about by the revolutions in computing and communications that are shrinking the globe, allowing access to knowledge and to markets for people who had previously been denied it by circumstance or hierarchy.

It may be that, like the outbreak of the Great War in 1914, this is the moment when the new century begins to confront itself and turns its back on the long boom that led up to the Millennium – just as the twentieth century turned away from the long Edwardian summer of the British Empire a century ago. As then, there are many tensions and frictions between countries and within countries. The old order is falling apart. Our ideas and our ways of looking at the world will change. We will be open to the new. The old institutions will become irrelevant and vanish.

Whatever happens, we know from history that it will undoubtedly be a very long and difficult process of change as people and nations give up cherished ideas, assumptions and habits and make way for the new. We seem destined for what the Chinese curse calls 'interesting times'.

We can see how important the concept of global health is within this much wider context both because it will affect everything else and because it is affected by everything else. Progress in low- and middle-income countries, as we will see, will depend in part on changing the pattern of international relationships that contribute to their problems. Richer countries share their vulnerabilities but are also confronted by the increasingly obvious fact that western scientific medicine, whilst science and technology will bring great benefits, cannot cope by itself with the problems of the future and needs to adapt and evolve to survive.

The position is very similar to where we were before the credit crunch shattered our ideas about finance. Our bubble of raised expectation, of hope and hype, is bursting before our eyes. We are heading for a health crunch: the meeting of the unsustainable past with the unknowable future.

In a crisis it is often the new ideas and innovations that will be the most important. In recession businesses that innovate with their eyes on the opportunities of the future are the ones that succeed. In health we need to do the same. We already know that it is very likely that we are going to be poorer in the future and need to spend more effort on prevention of disease and promotion of health. We need to find the new ideas that will help us be successful in this future environment and to learn from those who already have to think in this way.

It is the ideal moment to try to learn from the poor and disadvantaged rather than to go backwards to the habits and thought patterns of the past.

Turning the world upside down

Not everything is gloomy or depressing in poor countries. Several countries in Southeast Asia have prospered enormously in recent years. Developing countries and emerging markets in South America and eastern Europe have, until the credit crunch at least, seen growth. Sub-Saharan Africa grew at 4% a year from 2004 to 2008, a faster rate than Europe, and experienced fewer wars and harboured fewer tyrants than there were 10 years ago,[16] giving grounds for hope for the future. In all these countries, as we have seen with BRAC, people are innovating and creating new solutions to their problems.

There is another way of looking at the world in which we turn it upside down and ask what would it be like if the import–export business in health workers and ideas described earlier were reversed and poorer countries exported their ideas and experience whilst richer ones exported their health workers?

Some months before I visited Bangladesh, I had been in Ethiopia, where I met a young British Consultant, Dr Martin Beed. He was working in Jimma University Hospital in southern Ethiopia for a short period as part of a partnership scheme with Nottingham University Hospital in the UK. Every year for the last 15 the hospitals had been exchanging small groups of staff for up to a month at a time. The original idea and still the main purpose was to help train and educate health workers in the Jimma Hospital both in Jimma itself and on their visits to the UK. Increasingly, however, it had become obvious that the British people also benefited, learning about Ethiopia and about themselves at the same time.

Jimma University Hospital is fairly typical of the larger old African hospitals with a few modern buildings of three or four stories, used mostly by the University, surrounded by mainly single story wards and departments. It was in reasonable repair, although the concrete blocks, bare plaster and curtainless windows contrasted sharply even with Nottingham's oldest buildings at home. It was close to the countryside and on one occasion as we spoke there were monkeys jumping on and off the roof, their faces appearing momentarily at the windows of the ward before being shooed away by the staff and visitors.

I asked Dr Beed why he was there. He told me that one of the reasons he had wanted to come on the scheme was because there had been a large increase in TB where he worked in Nottingham. There had been five cases in the Intensive Care Unit in the last year and he wanted to go somewhere where they understood the disease well and he could gain more experience of it.

In the event he had learned about TB, but he had also been surprised to see that the local staff had such good clinical skills, better than many, if not most, UK doctors. By this he meant that, in the absence of all the equipment, nurses and doctors needed to look at the patient properly, talk to them, assess the feel and texture of their skin and pulse and make a clinical judgement from their verbal and other responses. All this had to be done without the instruments British doctors would have relied on at home.

I asked what else had surprised him in Ethiopia. He told me that he was teaching on a direct entry anaesthetics course, where people with high school education were trained to use a range of anaesthetics after 4 years' training. This is very uncommon in the UK or other rich countries, yet it is the backbone of the anaesthetic service in many Sub-Saharan African countries. We generally require full medical training before anyone can give anaesthetics.

Moreover, he had been intrigued to see the way that education in Jimma University was so entirely community based. At every stage and at every opportunity, students of every discipline from agriculture to health care were linked to local communities and learned their profession and skills in the field rather than in the classroom.

As Dr Abraham Haileamlak, the Vice President for Clinical Service at Jimma University explained, he wanted to train people who could and would practice in the real conditions of rural Ethiopia. The three Medical Schools in Addis Ababa, he told me, used American curricula and turned out doctors better suited to emigrate than to work in their own country. Here in Jimma he trained them for their own country.

These things challenged our pre-conceived ideas. Dr Beed and I could have seen all this as just being a sad story of students who didn't have proper equipment and facilities and who were therefore being forced to learn, inadequately, from what was at hand. We didn't see it like that at all; although we knew of course that more money, more people and more equipment would make an enormous difference.

We realised that we were meeting able people who were getting a good grounding in their professions by learning from their patients and their communities as well as from their professors. We saw, too, that their education was based on knowing what was needed locally. It was based on their context and their circumstances. As Dr Beed put it in a later article: "Although resource-poor, the medical staff were far from knowledge-poor".[17]

There may have been bare plaster on the walls and monkeys on the roof, but these were very rich and challenging ideas for us to think about. Perhaps we should take them home with us and see how they could be applied there.

We can find, if we only try to look, many more examples where richer countries can learn from importing the ideas and experience of poorer countries. In countries as different as India and Uganda, health leaders are using the natural strengths of their countries, the sense of community and family and the desire for self-determination, to promote health and provide healthcare. They are supporting their women as the natural health leaders, linking microfinance schemes and health insurance and finding ways to reconcile local traditional medicine and its practitioners with the western scientific tradition.

There is no shortage of ideas and examples to copy. In Brazil, Mozambique and elsewhere governments are educating health workers to meet the needs of the country and not just of the professions. Local health workers, often called clinical officers, are trained in 3 years to deal with specific tasks such as undertaking caesarean sections or cataract operations, which require a full professional education elsewhere. Meanwhile, as we shall see later, New York City is already emulating Mexican policies to promote health education and international good practices in conditions as different as HIV/AIDS and club-foot that have been developed from experience in Africa.

On the other side of the import–export business there is a long and valuable tradition of partnerships between hospitals and communities in richer and poorer countries and many individuals have gone as paid workers, researchers and volunteers, individually or through organized schemes, to work in poorer countries. They and the country can both benefit.

There are thousands of health workers in rich countries who would gladly offer their skills to poor countries if the circumstances were right. They could support local people and institutions, train thousands more health workers in their own countries and help transform the lives of whole populations. Groups from the diaspora, the migrants themselves and their children, are also keen to help.

In return they would learn for themselves how to see their own world differently and to challenge the old assumptions of the industrialized health systems. Poorer countries, precisely because they have so few resources, have to learn how to engage patients and communities in their own care, how to prioritise promoting health over tackling illness, how to deploy new technologies effectively and how to manage the ever-growing burden of costs. These are exactly the sorts of issues that need to be grasped in richer countries as they come to terms with the diseases and long-term conditions of the twenty-first century. There is much that they might learn from experience in these poorer countries.

I have been very struck by the way that leaders in poorer countries, without either having the resources or being burdened by the established practices of the rich countries, have created new approaches and new ways of dealing with old problems. It is equally evident that many health workers from richer countries who find themselves dealing with patients in poorer countries without all their usual resources frequently find different ways of doing things. They learn for themselves and, if their home country were more receptive, might bring these ideas back home to great effect.

I have also been impressed by the way that many young health professionals, the students, doctors, nurses and others that I have met in the UK and the USA, see their careers very differently from their parents' generation and are nurturing new ideas and approaches. Whilst their elders are pre-occupied by running complex health systems and struggling to work out how to pay for all the new high-tech and high-cost treatments that industry can develop, the young professionals are interested in global health and in how society, the economy and the environment shape our health and our lives.

Both groups, the leaders in poor countries and the young professionals in the rich, are creating a new way of thinking about health. They are developing a new and explicitly global outlook that recognizes our interdependency and its implications but also stresses the uniqueness of each situation and the way that the local blend of social, political, economic and environmental circumstances affect health.

This approach respects evidence and science, but wants to understand how things get done in practice and what role patients and the public play alongside scientists and clinicians. It doesn't start, as western medical education has traditionally done, by studying the science and then applying it to society but, rather, turns the world upside down and starts with understanding society and seeks to apply the findings from both the natural and the social sciences. It is a profound difference that influences the way that clinicians think and behave.

This approach of learning from the poor, the young and the excluded when combined with the new sciences and technologies – where the Internet and the contraceptive pill have already turned our world upside down – will help us confront and tackle the challenges of the future.

My ideas had also been challenged, earlier, in the totally different circumstances of the USA, where the rich, at least, can have the benefits of every sort of equipment, facility and medication. There I met doctors and scientists who are able to chart our genetic makeup and pinpoint with extraordinary accuracy the vulnerable areas where disease could attack and take hold. Personal medicine with drugs and therapies tailored to our precise needs is now becoming a reality. The Internet already has many sites where you can have your genes analysed, read the runes about your chances of Alzheimer's or diabetes and learn about, plausible or implausible, ways of trying to avoid your fate.

As our search returns to richer countries we can see the great advances in science, computing and communications, the accompanying progress in personalised medicine and the way in which systems thinking is helping improve the safety and quality of healthcare. Many examples from the USA and from my own experience in the NHS illustrate the great potential in these areas but also reveal the ethical and practical problems they can bring.

There is a great deal of technology, knowledge and basic resources that need to be transferred from the rich world to the poor if the health of the poorest is to be improved. However, at the same time and partly due to their very poverty, pioneers and leaders in poor countries are developing new ideas and new approaches to health that may have real relevance and application in rich countries. We can all learn from each other.

We can also see in richer countries how disability campaigners, social entrepreneurs and community activists are using concepts of human rights and responsibilities to challenge traditional thinking and re-design services. They provide interesting parallels with activity and activists in poorer countries working towards self-help and self-determination.

This exploration of examples and experiences around the world allows us to start to identify the practical knowledge of people and societies, science and systems that will be necessary for the future: the twenty-first-century knowledge that will equip our health workers and ourselves to address the needs of the twenty-first century. They no longer need to work with the ideas and tools of the twentieth century.

The paradigm shift towards global health

Many young health professionals appear to have an instinctive understanding of the changes taking place, with thousands of them signing up to organisations and courses on global health. Leaders in many poorer countries have embraced changes in their own policies and actions. Individual pioneers are running projects and programmes, large and small, which embody the changed way of looking at the world.

The authorities of the old system, the vested interests that keep it in place may not see it, but the world is shifting around them. There is a movement of people and of ideas and, as we explore further, we can begin to see that global health truly opens the way to a paradigm shift with three distinct strands.

It is, firstly, concerned with independence and self-determination. Personal, cultural and social issues determine what people value and how they want to live their lives and manage their health. Health is no longer seen simply as the absence of disease or a sense of wellbeing, but as independence and the ability to live lives we have reason to value, whether we are rich or poor, old or young, disabled or dying. We want our lives back when we are ill, we want to retain our independence when we are old and we want to be the judges of our own quality of life.

Secondly, it is based on our interdependence and on mutuality. It values the contributions of laypeople alongside professionals and public sector alongside private, and stresses the importance of family and community, with the leading role of women at its heart. It embraces the understanding that when rich and poor countries work together both gain. Benefits are mutual. There are opportunities for shared learning and co-development.

Thirdly, it embodies the belief that health is a basic human right and that people are entitled to expect their governments to safeguard and promote their health just as they expect them to defend the country and ensure public safety, the education of children and economic stability. This is accompanied by a demand for greater openness and accountability at every level of authority. We no longer take everything on trust. We want to see the evidence.

These three strands are forcing a shift in the way the core features of western scientific medicine – greater professional competence, scientific discovery, commercial innovation and massive spending – operate in practice.

All these core features are turned upside down as part of this paradigm shift:

- Greater professional competence is achieved through patients and communities empowering and working with professionals.
- Scientific discovery is made relevant by our understanding of society and of how to apply it.
- Commercial innovation is effective only as part of wider goals.
- Measures of input spending are replaced by measures of the social and economic value achieved.

The search for global health in the twenty-first century

Turning the World Upside Down follows the pattern of my own search for understanding. The first two chapters look at poorer countries and richer countries in turn, providing the background, facts and figures and basic analysis that set the context for the rest of the book. They are, inevitably, the most dense and slowest part of the book to read, but help make sense of what follows.

In the next three chapters I deal with the relationships between poorer and richer countries and tackle some of the more controversial questions about migration, the value of aid, and what we in the rich West can learn from people in Africa, Asia and Latin America.

The following three chapters begin to pull all our learning together. They describe the work of pioneers and innovators from around the world in order to illustrate the sort of practical knowledge we are going to need to tackle the problems of the twenty-first century successfully. They show how there is a shift in the paradigm of western scientific medicine. The old model developed in the nineteenth and twentieth centuries isn't sufficient any more but has to adapt to the needs of today.

Finally, the last two chapters conclude by proposing a programme of action to accelerate the changes that are already underway in many parts of the world, make them more visible and more coherent and help to improve health globally. These ideas are only ideas until they are implemented and we can see what they mean in reality.

Throughout I have used examples and stories from my own experience and my own journey to describe what I have seen and learnt and to bring these ideas alive. I have had my old ideas challenged and changed by what I have seen and heard and I have been reminded that, whatever else is going on in the world, change needs to happen in the most important places of all – our minds, our beliefs and our behaviours.

References

1. Crisp N. *Global Health Partnerships: The UK contribution to health in developing countries.* 2007. Available at: www.dh.gov.uk/en/Publicationsandstatistics/Publications/PublicationsPolicyAndGuidance/DH_065374.
2. UNICEF. *Reduce child mortality.* [Online]. Available at: www.unicef.org/mdg/childmortality.html.
3. *The Millennium Development Goals Report 2008.* United Nations Organisation. Available at: www.un.org/millenniumgoals/pdf/The%20Millennium%20Development%20Goals%20Report%202008.pdf.
4. *World Trade Report 2006.* World Trade Organisation. Available at: www.wto.org/english/res_e/booksp_e/anrep_e/wtr06-1a_e.pdf.
5. Dowden R. *Obama's direct line to the heart of Africa.* The Times. 10 July 2009 p31.
6. Crump L, Maswood SJ. *Developing Countries and Global Trade Negotiations.* Oxford: Routledge, 2007.
7. Land deals in Africa and Asia: Cornering foreign fields. *The Economist.* [Online] 21 May 2009. Available at: www.economist.com/opinion/displaystory.cfm?story_id=13697274. [Accessed 17 September 2009].
8. Chen L, Narasimhan V. *Health and human security: Pointing a way forward.* Available at: www.fas.harvard.edu/~acgei/Publications/Chen/LCC_Health_and_HS_way_forward.pdf.
9. *Anti-tuberculosis Drug Resistance in the World.* World Health Organization. 4, 2008. Available at: whqlibdoc.who.int/hq/2008/WHO_HTM_TB_2008.394_eng.pdf.
10. Gray M. Climate change is the cholera of our era. *The Times* [Online] 25 May 2009. Available at: www.timesonline.co.uk/tol/comment/columnists/guest_contributors/article6355257.ece.
11. Costello A, Abbas M, Allen A et al. Managing the health effects of climate change. Lancet and University of London Institute for Global Health Commission. *The Lancet* 2009; **373**: 1693–733.
12. Jay M, Marmot MG. *Health and climate change* (editorial). *BMJ* 2009; **339**: b3669. Available at: www.bmj.com/cgi/content/extract/339/sep15_1/b3669.
13. Jacques M. When China rules the world: The rise of the middle kingdom and the end of the western world. London: Allen Lane, 2009.
14. Hutton W. *The Writing on the Wall: Why We Must Embrace China as a Partner or Face it as an Enemy.* New York: Free Press, 2006.
15. Emmott B. *Rivals: How the Power Struggle Between China, India and Japan Will Shape our Next Decade.* Florida: Harcourt, 2008.
16. Dowden R. *Africa: altered states, ordinary miracles.* London: Portobello Books Ltd; 2008.
17. Beed M. Links with Ethiopia. *Anaesthesia News* [Online] 2009; **262**: 18–20. Available at: www.aagbi.org/publications/anaesthesia_news/2009/may09.pdf.

2 Health and poverty

"Take the death of this small boy this morning, for example. The boy died of measles. We all know he could have been cured at the hospital. But the parents had no money and so the boy died a slow and painful death, not of measles, but out of poverty."[1]

These words spoken by a man in Ghana show just how intimately poverty and ill health are linked together. Every year, 9.2 million children die before the age of 5; two-thirds of these deaths, 6 million, are preventable.[2] The leading causes of childhood deaths – pneumonia, diarrhoea, malaria and measles – are easily prevented with a few basic things such as clean water, insecticide-treated bed nets, oral rehydration and immunisations. All these diseases can be linked back to poverty.

Each of these children is an individual – someone's child; but sadly many do not have a mother or father to mourn them. A good part of a generation of adults in southern Africa has died of AIDS, leaving their children to fend for themselves or be cared for by already overburdened relatives and, sometimes, strangers. In India, where the Taj Mahal stands as a memorial to an Emperor's wife, Mumtaz Mahal, who died in childbirth in 1631, about 1 in 200 births still result in the death of the mother, whilst an equal number lead to painful injuries.[3] Their surviving children suffer with them.

This chapter continues the search to understand what is happening globally by asking why this is still happening. Why, after all the effort and the aid that has been put in by national governments, countless non-governmental organisation (NGOs), the World Health Organisation (WHO) and by so many donors is the situation still so dreadful?

The headlines

Low-income countries are not all the same, any more than rich ones are. Africa is not a single place, nor is South America or South Asia. Environment, culture and the economy all matter. There have been extraordinary successes in some countries, their economies and their populations thriving, and awful failures in others. Nevertheless, as I have discovered from visiting a number of countries and talking to many people, it is possible to paint a simple picture that describes many of the problems faced in most of the poorer countries of the world.

There are two simple headlines and a third more complex one. Different observers may put more stress on one than the others, but in reality they are connected and all need to be addressed.

The first is that there is much more ill health, early death and disability in these countries than in richer ones and many more causes for the problems. Sub-Saharan Africa easily emerges as the region with the greatest problems. It has about 10% of the world's population but about 24% of all the disease. North America and Europe have between them about the same population but only about 5% of the disease.[4] Sub-Saharan Africa also has the widest range of problems. Communicable diseases like HIV/AIDS and malaria, non-communicable ones such as diabetes and heart failure, childbirth, war, violence and accidents all take their toll.

The second headline is that poverty and everything associated with poverty make matters worse and, of course, ensure that there aren't the resources to deal with any of the health problems properly. Health problems are reinforced and magnified by a wide range of factors associated with poverty including low levels of education, unstable societies, conflict, hunger, dirty water, bad nutrition, high birth rates, housing conditions, unemployment, crime, violence, unsafe working environments and, in some cases, corruption and the absence of the rule of law.

Poverty means that the poorest region of the world, Sub-Saharan Africa, has only 3% of the world's health workers and 1% of the world's health expenditure to cope with 24% of the world's burden of disease and ill health.[4] For individuals the costs of healthcare for themselves and their families can be catastrophic. The World Health Statistics Report 2008 calculates that over 100 million people are impoverished each year because they have to pay for healthcare.[3] Others simply don't get healthcare because of their and their country's poverty.

This takes us on to the third and more complex, and perhaps most controversial, headline. This is that national and international social, economic and political structures, between and within countries, generally keep the rich rich and the poor poor. They maintain the status quo.

We see this internationally, where richer countries by reason of historic power, alliances and, often, language and culture, occupy the powerful positions in international organisations from the Security Council to the World Bank and effectively determine the way international relationships work and business is conducted. As a result the terms of trade tend to favour rich countries and rich people to the disadvantage of low income countries and poorer citizens around the globe and even international aid, as we shall see in later chapters, comes with its own ideological and cultural baggage.

Prosperity is very fragile in many of these countries and people live their lives on the edge and are very dependent on others. To put it at its simplest, in countries where a single export dominates their economy, such as Zambia with copper or Haiti with sugar, a fall in world commodity prices can be disastrous.

The international situation is mirrored nationally where poorer people tend to be marginalized and excluded from decision making. They are often unable to help themselves, let alone secure the services they need. Cultural and social issues may generate tensions in some societies and family and tribal groups may dominate politics and the economy. These cultural and social issues as we shall see may have a very significant effect on health.

These differences between rich and poor, the haves and have-nots, which are visible enough even in rich countries, are magnified many times over in poorer countries where very often a small elite coexists with a large and very poor population with poorer education, worse nutrition and less opportunity to advance.

Many governments in poorer countries lack the checks and balances and accountability arrangements prevalent in longer established countries and corruption remains a major problem in many of them. Another quotation, this time from a man in eastern Europe, from *Voices of the Poor* shows that that this is not lost on poorer people. "What type of government do we have? One hand gives and the other takes away!"[1]

Low income countries and their poorest citizens are struggling against all the odds.

Success and achievement

Most of this chapter is devoted to looking at the problems that people face in poorer countries. It shows how the problems of health, poverty and society intersect at every level and how solutions need to address all three. It necessarily paints a gloomy picture.

It would be a mistake, however, to think that everything is awful. There are great successes to talk about, from the well-publicised growth of many Asian countries to the continuing rise of Latin American countries and the less well-known renaissance that is underway in Africa.[5] It would also be a mistake to think that further improvements are going to come mainly from aid and development support and the actions of richer countries and international organisations. In most cases change will come from within.

Turning the World Upside Down contains many stories of great leadership and achievement. There is evident innovation, activity and energy in almost every country and it is no surprise that authoritative figures like Francis Omaswa, who has played a leading role in Ugandan and global health organisations, talk of hope and of there never having been a better opportunity to make improvements. Africa, as well as Asia and America, is on the move. We need to see the problems in context. There have been substantial improvements over the years and we need to make sure that the sheer scale of the remaining problems doesn't disguise this fact or lead to unnecessary despondency about the possibility of improvement.

One of the remarkable features in recent years is how the world is coming together to address health and social issues and how health and development are now so high on the agenda at meetings of world leaders. Almost every country in the world has signed up to the Millennium Development Goals: committing themselves by 2015 to, amongst other things, stop the growth in HIV/AIDS, TB and malaria, reduce childhood deaths by two-thirds and reduce by three-quarters the number of mothers who die in childbirth or as a result of pregnancy.

The UN report published halfway through this period showed that progress had been made on the first two goals and that there is a reasonable chance of achieving them. The third one, concerning maternal mortality, is, however, falling well behind.[6]

There has been demonstrable progress with HIV/AIDS, TB and malaria. In 2007 the Global Fund calculated that 2 million people were now on anti-retroviral therapy,[7] which controls but does not cure AIDS, and that the number of new cases has been declining since 2000. In 2008, 100 million additional insecticide-treated bed nets to combat malaria were distributed worldwide[8] and US$4 billion has been invested in the search for vaccines for these and other diseases.[9] There has, similarly, been a significant improvement in child mortality in most countries in recent years. Bangladesh, for example, has reduced the mortality of the under 5s by 40% between 1990 and 2007, whilst global figures record a 35% fall.[10]

This progress comes against a background where life expectancy in low- and middle-income countries has increased faster than in high-income ones over the last 50 years, albeit from a lower base, where economies in many of these countries have been growing fast and where there have been successful campaigns in many parts of the world to tackle diseases such as cholera and polio.

Figure 2.1 shows how life expectancy at birth has changed between 1950 and 2005 in different regions of the world. Overall, much of the improvement has come from very big reductions in deaths amongst newborn and small children. The size of the regions does, however, mask big differences between countries; so for example, the worsening position in Russia and parts of eastern Europe disguises the high and growing life expectancy in the west of the region. Nevertheless, even at this scale, the size of the improvement in Asia and the Middle East is spectacular as is the widening of the gap between Africa and most of the rest of the world.

Between 1950 and 2005 life expectancy has increased by:

- 27 years in Asia to 68
- 23 years in Latin America and the Caribbean to 73*
- 23 years in the Middle East to 67
- 14 years in Oceania to 74
- 11 years in Sub-Saharan Africa to 49
- 9 years in North America to 78*
- 8 years in Europe to 74

Figure 2.1 Life expectancy in low- and middle-income countries has grown faster than in high-income countries between 1950 and 2005. From World Health Statistics 2009. From World Population Prospects, 2006 Revision, United Nations. New York, 2007, p19, ESA/P/WP.202

These substantial improvements have come from a mixture of action taken to improve health and the impact of economic growth and improved wealth. It has been estimated that half of the improvement observed in poorer countries resulted from growing wealth but that a significant part came from specific health interventions such as eliminating polio in Latin America and the Caribbean and controlling TB in China.[11]

Against this background of past success and of hope for the future, let us return to the problems of today.

The first headline – the burden of disease

Poorer countries simply have more disease than richer ones and more causes of ill health, disability and death. Here, we will look in a little more detail at what that means in practice and at how non-communicable diseases such as diabetes are becoming major problems, alongside communicable ones. We will also look at how women and children and people with disabilities are affected.

Figure 2.2, which shows the size of continents in terms of deaths from often preventable diseases, provides a simple visual illustration of where the main problems are. Africa and South Asia loom large, whilst the Americas and Europe shrink to relative insignificance. Sub-Saharan Africa, as was noted earlier has 10% of the world's population and 25% of the disease.

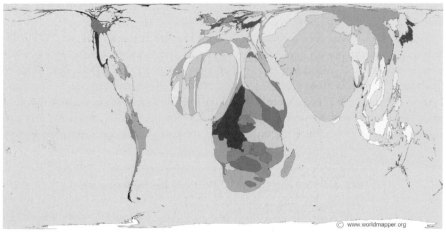

Figure 2.2 Distribution of often preventable deaths. From Worldmapper 2009. The size and shading of countries on the map reflects the scale of the problem

Communicable and non-communicable diseases

The communicable diseases such as HIV/AIDS, malaria and TB are still the biggest killers in Sub-Saharan Africa, whilst malaria and TB cause enormous suffering in parts of South Asia.

A few simple facts speak for themselves and illustrate the depth of the problem. Over 1 million people are killed worldwide by malaria every year; they are mostly children under the age of 5.[12] TB kills 1.7 million people each year.[13] HIV/AIDS has had an even more shocking impact in Sub-Saharan Africa. Life expectancy fell by 12 years in South Africa and 18 years in Swaziland between 1990 and 2005, largely due to HIV/AIDS.[3]

These figures help explain why Africa has seen such a relatively low increase in life expectancy compared to the rest of the world. Even now that progress has been made and new cases of HIV/AIDS are reducing, these diseases are not beaten. Prevalence of HIV/AIDS in South Africa remains very high at 18.3% in 2006.[14] There are new cases every year and the threat of multi-drug resistance in TB and malaria is on the horizon.

Even where these diseases are well managed and controlled, they complicate every other aspect of healthcare from childbirth to mental health. As Dr Molefi Sefularo, the South African Deputy Minister for Health, explained to me, they will remain the dominant factors in health system planning in every country that has been badly affected. The legacy of the HIV/AIDS epidemic will be with us for decades to come.

These major and widespread communicable diseases have caught the world's attention but there are others, some of which have been called the neglected tropical diseases, which are locally widespread and important. There are now 14 diseases, such as river blindness, sleeping sickness and leprosy, which have been officially classified as 'neglected tropical diseases' and all of which present significant problems, in part because they have been neglected. They affect about 1 billion people in the world but, as diseases of the poor they do not represent a good market for the drug developers nor have they been well researched by academics or understood by clinicians globally.

Communicable diseases have been, and remain, a dreadful scourge in Africa and elsewhere, but the growing problem is non-communicable disease. The biggest causes of death outside Africa are now the non-communicable diseases: and most significantly, diseases of the heart and vascular systems, cancers and diabetes.

These diseases tend to increase as populations grow richer and adopt new lifestyles with different diets and less physical activity. This is part of what academics call the epidemiological transition from diseases of the poor to the so-called 'diseases of affluence'.[15]

Figure 2.3 illustrates the impact of these diseases, not in terms of deaths, but in terms of the burden of disability they place on a country or a region. It is the burden of constant illness and suffering that weighs very heavily on individuals and their families and on the economy and functioning of their country. It shows very clearly that Sub-Saharan Africa and South Asia face a double problem of both communicable and non-communicable diseases and a high burden of disability caused by maternal, perinatal and nutritional causes. It also shows how big a burden non-communicable diseases place on Europe and Central Asia, in part reflecting the very unhealthy environment and lifestyles in the former USSR and its satellites.

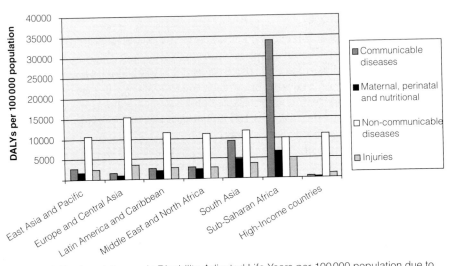

Figure 2.3 Burden of disease in Disability-Adjusted Life Years per 100 000 population due to broad disease categories by region for 2002. (The 'DALY' combines in one measure the time lived with disability and the time lost due to premature mortality.)

The very simplicity of the chart disguises the differences in the way diseases manifest themselves in different countries and their different consequences. Diabetes, which now affects 230 million people worldwide, most of whom live in low- or middle-income countries, is generally manageable in richer countries.[16] It can, however, quickly be fatal in poor countries, where it may go undiagnosed and where insulin may well not be available.

Delivering healthcare is very different in different parts of the world. The diseases and their presentation may be different. Complications need to be taken into account, where for example, expectant mothers have malaria or HIV/AIDS leads to mental illness. The availability of resources and the physical, social and cultural environments also affect what can be done. These factors tend to make it more difficult to deliver healthcare in poorer countries and mean that it is not possible simply to transfer the procedures and skills learned in wealthier countries to poorer ones. There is the need to understand the local context in all its aspects.

Professor Eldryd Parry who, although Welsh, has worked in African countries for more than 40 years, has developed a deep understanding of medicine in these environments and influenced many people, including me. Together with colleagues, he has written the definitive textbook on medicine in Africa, which places its practice firmly in the local context of the local diseases and their local manifestations, the local resources and the local culture.[17]

Reading it, one is left wondering if a similar volume is also needed in richer countries, where diseases, resources and culture may also be very different from the scientific norm. It is a point we will return to later in the book.

Women and children

Social and cultural issues come to the fore when we examine the health of women and children, who, in general, bear the greatest burdens in the poorest countries. This is partly due to the risks of childbirth and the sheer vulnerability of children. However, it is also about society and the way in which both women and children may be neglected in favour of feeding and looking after the adult males and the current and future breadwinners.

It has been estimated that there are 100 million fewer women in the world than you would expect, given the normal distribution of births and deaths. In South Asia, West Asia, and China, the ratio of women to men can be as low as 1 : 0.94 and it varies widely elsewhere in Asia, in Africa, and in Latin America.[18]

Part of this is due to poor nutrition and lack of healthcare. Many girls are given less food than boys and are less likely to receive healthcare. This leads to problems later in life, with under nourishment making childbirth more risky and increasing the susceptibility to a number of diseases. Matters are made worse by the preference for male children in some societies and, in some of them, the abortion of female foetuses and murder of female babies.[19]

These essentially social and cultural factors contribute very substantially to the fact that around half a million women die each year of pregnancy-related causes and a further

600 000 are injured. About 3 million children, born and unborn, also perish in the womb or shortly after birth.[20]

Mothers are essential for the healthy and safe upbringing of their children. Studies show that a mother's education also profoundly affects how likely her children are to live. Two multinational surveys showed that children of mothers with no education had 2.2 times higher mortality than those whose mothers had had education. They also showed that rural mortality was 1.5 times higher than urban, reflecting the different conditions and poorer access to education and services, and that poorer children overall had 2.5 times higher mortality.

Whilst there have been real improvements in the death rates of children, improvements in maternal health are, however, far too slow to achieve the targeted reduction of three-quarters by 2015. Figure 2.4 shows the distribution of these maternal deaths worldwide with the familiar pattern that the poorest regions of the world suffer most.

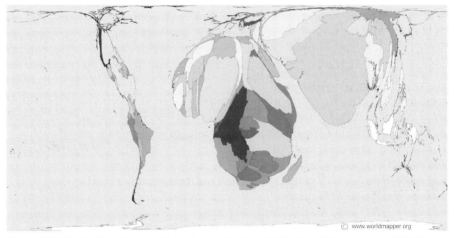

Figure 2.4 Distribution of maternal deaths worldwide in 2000. From Worldmapper 2009. The size and shading of countries on the map reflects the scale of the problem

Paradoxically, the world knows what it can do about this. The technical healthcare solutions to the problem are understood. Any of the major international agencies from United Nations Children's Fund (UNICEF) to United Nations Population Fund (UNFPA) can list the same small set of interventions that would deal with much of the problem. These include universal access to family planning, focused primary and antenatal care, attended delivery and postpartum care and access to emergency obstetric care.[17] The outstanding problems lie in the lack of resources and health systems needed to deliver this care and in the prevailing social and cultural attitudes.

One of the biggest resource problems is the lack of skilled birth attendants. Only 6% of mothers had a skilled health worker attend them at delivery in Ethiopia in 2002.[3] The average in Africa is less than 50%; the highest level in Africa was 99%, achieved in Mauritius.[3] In India it was 47%.[3] Anything less than 100% in rich countries would be regarded as shocking, unless the mother has specifically chosen to give birth without this support.

More generally, pregnant women need a health system that functions well across the whole range of services from community care to the most specialised hospital treatment if they are to thrive and survive. This means in practice that maternal health is the best indicator of the health of an entire health system and suggests that improving the system for pregnant women is likely to improve it for everyone else.

Underpinning everything are the social issues and the value placed on the lives of women and children. To take one simple example, in parts of Nigeria women cannot leave the house without the permission of their husbands and do not generally go to a clinic or hospital to give birth. Elsewhere women are expected to manage with the help of an untrained traditional birth attendant, as their mothers and grandmothers did. Their chances of surviving a problematic labour are massively reduced as a result.

Disability, damage and dependency

The scale and impact of disability in poorer countries can easily be overlooked by contrast with the drama of trying to save and treat people with high-profile diseases, yet it is a profound human and economic problem.

These very diseases add to the long-term problems of disability and dependency. The HIV/AIDS epidemic has produced thousands of people who are now weakened and dependent on drugs whilst malaria produces recurring bouts of sickness, and heart disease can cripple as well as kill. The reality of these diseases is very often poorer lives, stunted growth, lower resistance to other diseases and a reduced ability to earn a living.

Whilst some sorts of physical injury are often very visible, other types of disability are not. The millions of people depressed and stressed by illness or other causes, the people who are deaf or blind, the women damaged in childbirth and the thousands affected by the aftermath of illness may not be immediately obvious to an outside observer. There is social stigma attached to mental health and disability in many poor countries, just as there is in rich ones. The blind man, the disabled girl, the child unable to learn and the demented old woman are often hidden away in their own homes or kept out of sight in the family village.

Disability campaigners in rich countries have had to fight hard to get some level of equal treatment and to gain access to education and jobs as well as to services and buildings. Their counterparts in poor countries have an even greater struggle. The latest figures from the global campaign Education for All show, as one might expect, that 40 million of the 215 million children not yet in school are disabled.[21]

Local campaigners whom I spoke with in one Ugandan village had decided to do something about making disability both very visible and very audible. They started a disabled band and dance troupe. I watched them perform in exuberant style on a patch of land beside the local school. Blind performers, white sticks in hand, danced vigorously; whilst those unable to walk played instruments or sang. The schoolchildren dressed, boys and girls alike, in a bright pink uniform sang and danced around the edges. They allowed some people without disabilities to become part of the group and it had become a real institution in the area, a source of local pride as well as entertainment.

The performance over, I was taken to a single-roomed building that housed a branch of a microcredit bank that had been established specifically to cater for disabled people, although it too was open to others. Here, disabled people were able to save and to borrow money to start small ventures. The bank implicitly recognized that poverty can lead to disability and disability to poverty and had been established to help break the link locally. I later met blind men and women caring for animals and looking after crops who had been funded by the Bank. Disabled people can lead active lives and contribute to society.

Part of the tragedy is that so much of the disability as well as the disease could be prevented. A total of 800 000 people died as a result of injuries in Sub-Saharan Africa in 2001; 300 000 of these deaths were due to war and conflict, crime and violence. A further 200 000 died as a result of road accidents, due to the very poor driving and road conditions in the continent.[22] It is no surprise that so many vehicles in many African countries carry religious slogans such as In God We Trust and Trust No Other.

The other 300 000 deaths came from a wide range of causes in the home and employment. Whilst health and safety legislation may sometimes seem an unreasonable burden in rich countries, the absence of any such controls in most poor countries leads to a devastating toll of death and injury every year from falls from buildings, exposure to poisonous chemicals and mining. Physical trauma is one of the main causes of death in Africa and has enormous knock-on consequences.

As a result of the high level of disability, the percentage of dependent people to those able to work is about 10% in Sub-Saharan Africa and 7% elsewhere. In Sub-Saharan Africa a significant proportion of this is due to disability and illness amongst working-age people. In other parts of the world, where people live longer, dependency is more often due to age; this has a very big impact on the economic capability of the region as well as on the health and welfare of its inhabitants.

Disability and dependency have, perhaps not surprisingly, taken a lower priority than the immediate task of dealing with the big killer diseases. However, they will increasingly need to be the focus of attention and policy as the individual diseases are brought under control and renewed emphasis can be given to the overall health and productivity of the population.

These high levels of disability and dependence have a major economic impact. Poor health, poverty, disability and high birth rates all affect the economy. Conversely, improvements in health can have a significant impact on the economy.[23]

The physical and emotional capacity of a population and its scope for independent and productive activity will be a key for the future.

Health and poverty – the second headline

The earlier discussion has already brought out the close relationship between health and poverty and revealed that there are many wider factors in the environment that determine health. These linkages mean that health policies need to be integrated with others dealing with education, agriculture, employment and economic growth in order to make health improvements.

Between them these factors affect the health and prospects of millions of people. There is now clear evidence from many studies that reducing birth rates, improving education for girls, better nutrition, less crime and increased household incomes all contribute to improving health.[24] Whilst the absence of these factors can lead to a downward spiral of poor health and poor prospects, their presence can lead onwards and upwards to better things. Figure 2.5 illustrates this.

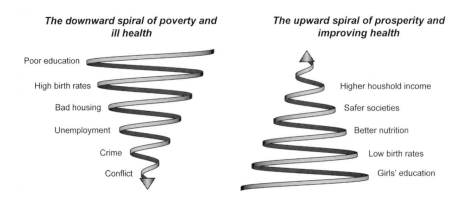

The downward spiral of poverty and ill health

Poor education
High birth rates
Bad housing
Unemployment
Crime
Conflict

The upward spiral of prosperity and improving health

Higher houshold income
Safer societies
Better nutrition
Low birth rates
Girls' education

Figure 2.5 Relationship between health and poverty

Looked at in this way the crucial question becomes how to convert the downward spiral into an upward one so that health and other benefits flow towards those most in need. What can practically be done to achieve this?

Part of the answer seems fairly clear and involves a pragmatic and practical approach to health improvement. So much of the death, disease and disability seen in poor countries is preventable and a little knowledge, clean water, protection from mosquitoes, the adding of micronutrients to food and a small range of drugs could work wonders. This has been well understood for years and has led health policymakers and planners to focus on primary care and prevention, working across sectors and with people in their own communities to prevent and treat disease there rather than treating the fully developed disease in, often distant, hospitals.

The Alma Ata Declaration of 1978 enshrined this as international policy. It defined primary healthcare in very wide terms to include education about health, nutrition, safe water and sanitation, maternal and child healthcare, family planning, immunisation against major infectious diseases, prevention and control of local diseases, treatment of common diseases and injuries, and provision of essential drugs.[25] It was an integrated and essentially common sense approach.

The Commission on the Macroeconomics of Health, reporting in 2001, advocated the community-based provision of an essential package of care, very much in line with Alma Ata, that it costed at US$34 per person per year. This set out a plan for poor countries based on the best analysis and evidence available.[26]

Despite this long held understanding of the problems and this clear approach, progress has been slow and the decision makers in national governments and their development partners have not generally adopted the model in practice, although they may have paid lip service to it in principle. Instead there has been investment in hospitals and in disease-specific services that ignored this wider context.

In Zambia at one point in the 1990s more than half the country's health budget was being spent in the main Lusaka hospital. More recently, in 2007, 90% of donor aid in Zambia was directed towards priority diseases rather than to supporting general health services or primary care.[27] The Alma Ata and Macroeconomics models are not being followed.

A significant part of the problem relates to the assumptions inherent in western scientific medicine, which has become the dominant model amongst professionals, planners and politicians in most of the world, that good healthcare revolves around doctors, hospitals and technical treatments. It undervalues, as we shall discuss in the next chapter, the role of the community and family, lifestyles, culture and behavioural and social factors.

Poverty means that there is also a chronic shortage of resources of all kinds for health care and results in the inability to create effective health systems to deliver these improvements.

Poverty means that the poorest region of the world, Sub-Saharan Africa, has only 3% of the world's health workers and 1% of the world's health expenditure to cope with 24% of the world's burden of disease and ill health.[4] It would appear tiny on a world map that showed countries in proportion to the healthcare resources they consumed. Europe would be very large and North America vast, with over 25% of total expenditure for 5% of the world's population. Figure 2.6 shows the relationship between resources, the health workforce and the burden of health for the richest and poorest continents.

Perhaps the most significant shortage in poorer countries is of trained health workers who can bring their expertise and skills to bear on the problems. In many cases even a little knowledge can help prevent disease or save a life. The World Health Report for 2006 estimated that there was a shortage globally of 4.3 million health workers with, in the familiar pattern, the poorest countries experiencing the greatest shortages.[4]

This is evident everywhere in poor countries. At a meeting of African Health Ministers in 2006 the Honourable Marjorie Nguange from Malawi told me that she had three pharmacists in the country and wanted four; whilst the Tanzanian Minister said that the most effective thing the UK could do would be to provide him with nurse tutors. Others demanded compensation for the professionals they had trained at local expense who now worked in the UK.

This theme of staffing and migration is dealt with at length in Chapter 4, where I argue that the UK and other countries that have benefited by this migration should provide compensation by supporting training in these countries.

This shortage of staff manifests itself not just as a shortage of doctors, nurses and other clinical staff but is revealed in the absence of all the managerial, administrative, maintenance and logistical staff that are needed to keep a system going. It turned out when I questioned Minister Nguange that she wanted pharmacists to supervise the distribution of drugs. It was a logistical and stock management problem. Her Ministry bought drugs centrally but was

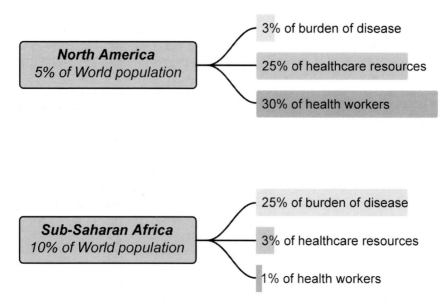

Figure 2.6 Comparison in burden of health and resources between the richest and poorest continents

unable to ensure their safe distribution with the result that drug cupboards in hospitals and clinics were all too often bare.

The problems of logistics, lack of maintenance of equipment, inadequate supply mechanisms and slow decision making are endemic in many poor countries. The position is further complicated by the way in which services are provided by a whole range of different providers – governments generally provide the basic service; whilst charities, international NGOs, traditional healers and others – contribute in different ways with very often little coordination or commonality of standards of quality. The fragmentation and unpredictability of services adds to the problems.

Underpinning these problems is the sheer shortage of money. The funding of health systems is a very complex issue in itself with a great deal of variation between countries. There are, however, a few general points that are worth drawing out here to help our understanding of the distinctive problems faced by low- and middle-income countries.

The starting point is that funding levels are very low compared to richer countries. The US spent US$6096 per head on health in 2006, whilst the UK spent US$2560. The difference between the lowest and highest spenders is enormous, with the 49 lowest income countries together spending US$31 billion per year, or US$25 per head, on the health of their 1.2 billion population in 2006. This is roughly equivalent to the money spent on the 6.5 million people living in the state of Arizona in the USA in the same year.[28]

An obvious question to ask would be how much more money is actually needed in the poorer countries of the world? What is the funding gap?

It is, however, much harder to estimate the amount of additional money needed to deliver improvements than to calculate current spend, partly for methodological reasons and partly because it depends on what improvement is being aimed for. The Taskforce on Innovative International Funding for Health Systems, reporting in July 2009, used two different methodologies to calculate what would be needed for the 49 lowest income countries to achieve the Millennium Goals. Under one scenario the US$31 billion current health spend would need to increase by a further US$36 billion in 2015 and by US$45 billion on the other.[28]

Their figures are not very different in suggesting a rise to between US$49 and US$60 per head to those produced by the Commission on the Macroeconomics of Health in 2001, when it estimated a need for US$34 per head to provide a basic set of community services. The difference appears to be in methodology, timing and objectives.

The two different Task Force models rest on different assumptions about levels of capital expenditure and staffing. These models illustrate the point that decisions need to be made by countries about what sort of health services they want. There is an obvious danger in the assumption that services and staffing structures in poorer countries should mirror those in richer ones, even when, as we shall see in the next chapter, the rich countries themselves are finding them hard to fund. We need here, as elsewhere, to turn the world upside down and look for other solutions.

The final question we need ask here about funding is: who pays? The answer for the 49 poorest countries is that, on average, 54% of expenditure comes from private sources with 45% from government funds. By far the largest part of the private expenditure, an average of 46%, is out-of-pocket expenditure by the individual. It is precisely this sort of expenditure that leaves the individual open, without government funding or insurance, to catastrophic costs from any illness.[28]

Figure 2.7 shows who pays and reveals that, even in Africa, external sources including direct aid only provide for around 11% of total expenditure. It also shows that Europe has by far the highest level of general government expenditure.

This brief discussion shows why it is so important to find ways to safeguard the individual against uncovered health cost as well as to increase the total funding available for health in these countries.

WHO region	Total expenditure on health as % of gross domestic product	General government expenditure on health as % of total expenditure on health	Private expenditure on health as % of total health expenditure	External resources for health as % of total expenditure on health
Africa	5.5	47.1	52.9	10.7
Americas	12.8	47.7	52.3	0.1
Southeast Asia	3.4	33.6	66.4	1.9
Europe	8.4	75.6	24.4	0.1
Eastern Mediterranean	4.5	50.9	49.1	2.0
Western Pacific	6.1	61.0	39.0	0.2

Figure 2.7 Regional levels of expenditure on healthcare (2006). From World Health Statistics 2009

The third headline – challenging the status quo

Discussion earlier in this chapter has already begun to bring out the ways in which national and international social, economic and political structures and processes affect health.

International institutions, relationships, trade and aid have been created by the richer countries and operate on the basis of their assumptions and preferences. Unsurprisingly, they maintain the status quo. We will explore the international position in some detail in Chapters 4 and 5, when we look at the so-called 'brain drain' of skilled workers from poorer to richer countries and at the ideas and ideology that rich countries export alongside their aid.

Here, we will only note how the different aspects mesh together so effectively, with richer countries sharing aspects of culture and history, creating treaties and alliances and raising capital and promoting trade between themselves. Each part works with the others as illustrated in Figure 2.8.

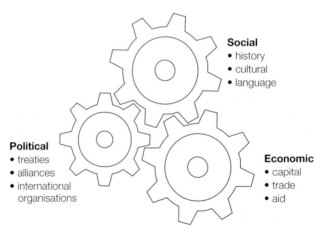

Figure 2.8 Social, political and economic structures work together to maintain the status quo

What happens within a society or a country is also very important. We have already noted how women's rights affect their access to healthcare, how a mother's education affects her children's chances of life and how social attitudes towards disabled people affect their opportunities at every turn. Health, education, tradition and legislation interact within every culture in a myriad different ways particular to the locality.

The Commission on the Social Determinants of Health undertook a very wide-ranging review of how social issues affect health, bringing together the facts and exposing the fictions. It analysed and described in considerable detail the ways in which social organisation, behaviours and structures determine the mental and physical health of individuals and groups in society. It showed, amongst other things, that there is a social gradient with a person's relative position in society affecting their chances of better or poorer health.

Its recommendations, published in 2008, were very straightforward. If we are really to be serious about improving health for everybody we must improve daily living standards and tackle the inequitable distribution of power, money and resources both nationally and internationally.[29] These recommendations explicitly address social, economic and political issues and have been seen by some people and governments as being far too partisan a political agenda. They take us into areas of social justice and rights that we will return to for further discussion in future chapters.

The commission's investigation of the evidence for links between economic growth and health is valuable, however, whatever the political context, in looking at whether it is sufficient simply to promote economic growth in order to improve health. It demonstrates that whilst economic growth is raising incomes in many countries, increasing national wealth alone does not necessarily increase national health. It depends how the wealth is used. It shows that there will not automatically be a 'trickle-down' effect to benefit the poor.

Some low- and middle-income countries such as Cuba, Costa Rica, China, the state of Kerala in India and Sri Lanka have achieved levels of good health despite relatively low national incomes. Others despite increased wealth have failed to improve the health of their whole populations.[29]

This demonstration is particularly important where health ministers have to argue hard within their government both for increased expenditure on health and for their share of the proceeds of growth. Countries need health infrastructure and spending as well as other public infrastructure. Free markets and economic growth will not simply provide for the millions still living in poverty.

Turning to government and governance, it is a sad fact that government in low-income countries can often be a byword for corruption, bureaucracy and disorganisation. The rhetoric of democracy, accountability and good governance all too often does not match the reality for both economic and social reasons. The Kenyan writer Binyavanga Wainaina describes the problem by saying: "We are often guilty of using words like leadership, government, parliament and institutions as if they represent solid realities … But in truth, all these structures are about as solid as free floating gases … we watch our Government float above us like a helium balloon tethered by the flimsiest of strings".[30]

Many countries simply do not have the resources and infrastructure or the outlook and culture necessary to hold governments and officials to account and make these institutions work effectively. Democracy and, in particular, democratic elections are extremely expensive and, more generally, all the apparatus of good government and accountability does not come cheap. Paul Collier, the author of *The Bottom Billion*, goes further and argues that elections can be counterproductive with autocrats learning to bribe, intimidate and cheat their way into power. They may gain themselves extra time in power as a result of their fraudulent election.[31]

Creating good governance and government is a very long-term process for any country. Outsiders may help, but the leadership must come internally. There have been improvements with regards to corruption in recent years. Transparency International, which has for years provided a country-by-country rating of corruption, the World Bank's global governance indicators and the more recent Ibrahim Index all show an improving trend.

Another positive indicator is that between 1960 and 1992, the period immediately after most countries became independent from the colonial powers, only three heads of state in Africa relinquished power voluntarily; since 1992, 40 have done so. It is a very big change; although examples such as Zimbabwe today show there is still further to go.

Governance and corruption remain very significant issues. As I write, several serving and former Kenyan Ministers are being accused of corruption and the Zambian Ministry of Health is under investigation for allegedly using health department money to support the government campaign for re-election.

We need however to be careful to understand how culture and family and ethnic links shape behaviour. In many poorer countries family loyalties are very important; elsewhere communities are the first loyalty for many people. Outsiders need to be careful about imposing their own values on how societies behave. There are, of course, some clear boundaries between corruption and normal cultural behaviour. Theft, bribery and demanding money with menaces are clear crimes, whilst networking, making friends and building alliances are natural and reasonable ways of behaving in any society. Cronyism and family ties operate in grey territory.

The boundaries of what constitutes reasonable behaviour are constantly shifting in all societies. There is an increasing expectation, in richer countries at least, that more and more decisions, from the size of an ex-banker's pension and the amount of MPs' expenses to the evidence used to go to war, should be open to public scrutiny. In the USA President Obama has had enormous difficulty in getting his appointees approved by Congress because all too many of them have in some way transgressed acceptable behaviour.

A look back into the history of any of today's rich countries will show us governments and societies that became rich and powerful through means and methods they would now disown and that economic growth and democracy did not always go hand in hand.

Leaders from poorer countries understand these issues very well and have had to face up to and fight corruption throughout their lives. I recall watching the Honourable Professor Sheila Tlou, then Minister of Health in Botswana, berate colleagues at a meeting about stamping out corruption. They couldn't blame the richer countries or expect them to tolerate it, she said. "No excuses, we have to deal with it", she said. She was not prepared to be a victim.

In January 2009 I asked a senior African leader what the election of a man of partly Kenyan heritage to the Presidency of the USA meant for Africa and Africans. "It's great…", he said and paused for maximum effect, "and now we have to behave ourselves!"

Three levels for action on health

This chapter has described three levels of problems and showed that health improvement needs to be tackled through confronting the health issues themselves, through alleviating poverty and through changing some of the social, political and economic structures that maintain the status quo.

In my exploration of these issues I have met people who advocate dealing with only one level of these problems saying, for example, that unless the world's trade relationships are sorted out, nothing else matters or that all we can do is offer practical help with health problems or that economic growth is the answer.

The truth is that these problems need to be tackled together to have greatest effect. Many countries have drawn up national development plans and poverty reduction plans that attempt to balance action in each of these areas. Figure 2.9 offers an example of the sort of actions that countries are taking to improve health in the context of their overall development. It has been put together from real examples from a number of different countries.

In creating this figure I have used the word *wealth* rather than *poverty* for the central column to indicate the ambition of all countries to grow their economy and increase the wealth of the country and its citizens.

The first level, tackling disease and ill health directly, is the most straightforward. At this level practically every government in the world recognizes health as one of its priorities alongside economic development, education and security. Most governments have established a national health system and have plans to improve the health of their populations. Most draw on learning and advice from elsewhere in doing so. Internationally, there are many examples of concerted efforts to improve health, ranging from dealing with particular diseases and their impact to developing drugs and vaccines for the diseases that primarily affect poor people and that the market would not otherwise fund.

The second level, creating wealth and tackling poverty in a country and dealing with its wider impacts, is more complex. At this level national governments take on all the

Health	Wealth	Society
Free access to basic healthcare services	Identification of and support for child headed households	Promotion of the private sector
Improve cross-sectoral cooperation for health promotion and public health	Implementing pro-poor policies	Development of ICT infrastructure and knowledge
Increase total government spending to 12% of GDP	Agricultural reform: facilitation of agricultural inputs and access to markets	Tax reforms
Increase numbers of trained health workers and improve retention measures	Food security	Enforcement of anti-corruption measures
Restructuring of National HIV/AIDS Council and implement 5-year strategic plan	Social action fund to support and finance the implementation of productive community and development programmes	Reform of the financial sector and the development of microfinance schemes
Increase immunisation coverage by 85%	Slums upgrading and low-cost housing	Reform of the security forces
Reduce under-5 mortality to 100/100 000 by 2010	Structural reform of water and sanitation services; expansion to urban poor and rural communities	Attainment of universal primary education
Reduce maternal mortality to 400/100 000 by 2010	Accelerate the pace of rural electrification programmes	Mainstreaming special groups into employment, e.g. women
		Rehabilitation and construction of the road network

Figure 2.9 Three levels for action on health

aspects of poverty, often through wide-ranging national poverty action plans, and work to promote economic growth amongst poorer communities. Internationally there are many examples of concerted efforts to reduce poverty through agricultural innovations and economic interventions.

The third level of action, tackling the status quo internationally and nationally, is however much more complex and problematic. It might seem as if this is purely a political matter with a need for the redistribution of power and wealth to create a fairer world and a level playing field. It is much more than this, however, involving as it does social, technological and economic changes that would not just flow from political change. It is not just government that needs to take the lead. Social leadership and advocacy of the sort necessary to change attitudes towards disabled people, promote their education and potential, and to change the way women are allowed to receive help at childbirth are necessary.

Economic and technological changes are vital with markets opened up and new technologies enabling people to participate in them and extend their potential. Mobile phones and computing bring social change as well as opportunity. The communications and Internet pioneers have enabled reform and the levelling of the playing field – the creation of a *flat world* that extends opportunity – in ways that social reformers and development workers could not dream of.[32]

Leadership

National and local leadership and political will are crucially important to making any such improvements. The implementation of these plans and long-term sustainable growth depends on local leadership and ownership.

In the research for *Scaling up, Saving Lives*, a report on how to improve and increase the training and education of health workers in low-income countries that I co-chaired with Bience Gawanas of the African Union, we looked at the evidence of what had worked in successful scale-ups around the world. The evidence was unequivocal: the most significant factor in every case was long-term sustained local political leadership.[33]

Foreigners can and do draw up excellent theoretical plans for improving health and health systems but they won't work unless national and local leaders embrace them and implement them. Technological improvements can be significant, but they can only work to their full extent where countries and leaders accept and adapt them to their own cultures and environments.

International organisations from donor countries to the World Bank and the WHO and international NGOs all have a part to play in support of the local leadership, wherever this exists. There is, as we shall see in Chapter 5, a great deal of controversy about exactly what role these external organisations can and should play and a great deal of questioning about the value of aid and international development.

This international dimension also needs to recognise our increasing interdependence in the face of spreading disease, the movement of populations, climate change and economic interconnectedness. The health of the world depends now more than ever on the strength of every country. New diseases will find the most vulnerable places to incubate and multiply before they spread. We are in this together. The health of poorer populations concerns us all.

Self-determination and self-help

It can be very easy in writing about health and poverty to discuss the actions of governments and business and international agencies and to ignore completely the experience and the potential of people who are themselves poor. As people from Georgia and Pakistan have said:

> *"Poverty is humiliation, the sense of being dependent on them, and of being forced to accept rudeness, insults, and indifference when we seek help."*[1]
>
> *"We poor people are invisible to others – just as blind people cannot see, they cannot see us."*[1]

In India I met the members of URVAL, a remarkable weavers' cooperative in the Thar Desert in Western Rajasthan, who have set up health and education programmes as well as providing income and employment for local people. The cooperative members want to be self-determining, in control of their lives and able to design their own route out of poverty. URVAL has a very powerful vision: "to lead the poor towards self-reliance by making available to them a package of development services that they themselves decide on, design, implement and eventually finance."

This example and others I describe later from the Kahnawake people in northern Canada and from Asia and Africa show groups and communities taking the future into their own hands. People whoever they are, whether they are rich or poor, sick or well, disabled or able bodied want to be heard and listened to, they want to be involved in decision making and they want to be seen for who they are and not for who we imagine they are. They also want justice and fair treatment.

These examples illustrate the themes of potential and possibilities and of justice and self-determination that run throughout the book and help shape both my observations and my conclusions. Ultimately, I believe, these themes will help create the solutions that we all want.

Conclusions

This chapter has provided an overview of health in poor countries as background and a starting point for the arguments that come later in *Turning the World Upside Down*. It offers a glimpse of the richness and variety of different experiences in different countries.

Each country is different and so is each community within it. There is good and bad. There are wonderful achievements and appalling crimes, great leaders and awful politicians. There are similarities and contradictions. There is great enterprise and there are appalling systems. Rich countries do good in poor countries and they do harm. There are no simple answers.

This chapter has introduced ideas about the importance of the social, political and economic context and the significance of disability and dependency that are as relevant in rich countries as in poor as we shall see in the next chapter.

It has also argued that efforts to improve health need to tackle problems at all three levels simultaneously – dealing clinically with disease, tackling poverty and disadvantage, and confronting the social, economic and political structures that get in the way of the solutions. Doing one without the others will only have limited impact.

The chapter raises the questions for later discussion of how international organisations can most effectively contribute towards improving health in poorer countries and of what impact the examples mentioned here of self-help and self-determination may have in the future.

Our search for understanding continues in the next chapter by looking at the current and past experience of richer countries: health and wealth.

References

1. Narayan D, Patel R, Schafft K, Rademacher A, Koch-Schulte S. *Voices of the Poor: Can Anyone Hear Us?* The World Bank. New York: Oxford University Press, 2000.
2. UNICEF. *Young Survival and Development*. [Online]. Available at: www.unicef.org/childsurvival/index. html.
3. World Health Organisation. *World Health Statistics 2009*.
4. World Health Organisation. *Working Together for Health. The World Health Report 2006*.
5. Dowden R. *Africa: Altered States, Ordinary Miracles*. London: Portobello Books Ltd, 2008.
6. The World Bank. *Global Monitoring Report 2009: A Development Emergency*. Available at: web. worldbank.org/WBSITE/EXTERNAL/EXTDEC/EXTGLOBALMONITOR/EXTGLOMONREP2009/ 0,,contentMDK:22149019~pagePK:64168445~piPK:64168309~theSitePK:5924405,00.html.
7. The Global Fund. *Global Fund Progress Report 2008*. Available at: www.theglobalfund.org/documents/ publications/progressreports/ProgressReport2008_ExecutiveSummary_en.pdf.
8. The Global Fund. *The Global Fund Annual Report 2008*. Available from: www.theglobalfund.org/ documents/publications/annualreports/2008/AnnualReport2008.pdf.
9. GAVI Alliance. *Cash received by GAVI at end of December 2008*. Available at: www.gavialliance.org/ resources/Donations_to_GAVI_2000___2008.pdf. [Accessed 28 September 2009].
10. UNICEF. *The State of the World's Children*. 2009. Available at: www.unicef.org/sowc09/index.php.
11. Levine R. and the What Works Working Group. *Millions saved-proven successes in global health*. Center for Global Development 2004.
12. World Health Organisation. *World Malaria Report 2008*. Available at: apps.who.int/malaria/wmr2008/ malaria2008.pdf.
13. World Health Organisation. *Global Tuberculosis Control – Surveillance, Planning, Financing*, 2008. Available at: www.who.int/tb/publications/global_report/2008/en/index.html.
14. UNAIDS. *South Africa: country situation*. [Online]. Available at: www.data.unaids.org/pub/FactSheet/ 2008/sa08_soa_en.pdf. [Accessed August 2009].
15. Ezzati M, Vander Hoorn S, Lawes CMM et al. Rethinking the 'diseases of affluence' paradigm: Global patterns of nutritional risks in relation to economic development. *PLoS Med* 2005; **2**: e133. Available at: doi:10.1371/journal.pmed.0020133.
16. World Diabetes Foundation. Available at: www.worlddiabetesfoundation.org/composite-35.htm.
17. Parry E, Godfrey R, Mabey D, Gill G. *Principles of Medicine in Africa*. 3rd edition. Cambridge: Cambridge University Press, 2004.
18. Sen A. More than 100 million women are missing. *The New York Review of Books*. Dec 20 1990; **37**(20). Available at: ucatlas.ucsc.edu/gender/Sen100M.html.
19. Barker D. *Nutrition in the Womb*. The Barker Foundation. 2008
20. UNICEF. *The State of the World's Children 2009*.
21. The World Bank. *Education for All: including children with disabilities*. 2003. Available at: siteresources. worldbank.org/DISABILITY/Resources/280658-1172610312075/EFAIncluding.pdf.
22. International Bank for Reconstruction and Development/The World Bank. 2006. *Global Burden of Disease and Risk Factors*. Washington: The World Bank and Oxford University Press.
23. Jamison DT, Bloom DE et al. *Health, health policy and economic outcomes*. UCLA Centre for Pacific Rim Studies, Los Angeles, CA. 1998.

24. World Bank. *World Development Report 2000/2001: Attacking poverty.* World Bank and Oxford University Press. 2001.

25. World Health Organisation. *Declaration of Alma Ata.* International Conference on Primary Health Care, Alma-Ata, USSR, 6–12 September 1978. The International Conference on Primary Health Care, 1978. Available at: www.who.int/hpr/NPH/docs/declaration_almaata.pdf.

26. World Health Organisation. *Macroeconomics and Health: Investing in health for economic development.* Report of the Commission on Macroeconomics and Health, 2001.

27. Update on the International Health Partnership and related initiatives (IHP+). Prepared for the Health 8 Meeting, 28 January 2008, Geneva.

28. Taskforce on Innovative International Financing for Health Systems. *More Money for Health and More Health for Money,* 2009. Available at: www.internationalhealthpartnership.net/pdf/IHP%20Update%2013/Taskforce/Johansbourg/Final%20Taskforce%20Report.pdf.

29. World Health Organisation. *Closing the Gap in a Generation: Health equity through action on the social determinants of health.* Commission on Social Determinants of Health, 2008.

30. Quoted by the Earl of Sandwich in House of Lords. Hansard 5 March 2009.

31. Collier P. More coups please. *Prospect* 26 April 2009; 157.

32. Friedman TL. *The World is Flat: A Brief History of the 21st Century.* New York: Farrar, Straus and Giroux, 2005.

33. Global Health Workforce Alliance. *Scaling Up, Saving Lives,* 2008.

3 Health and wealth

She was 19 and dying.

A healthy young woman, she had caught a virus which, by a one in a million chance, had attacked the heart muscle cells and she was now close to death from heart failure.

The situation was dire. Although drugs could damp down the inflammation, there wasn't enough time for them to work. The doctors treating her knew that if she could only survive for 48 hours the infection would be brought under control and her heart would start to recover. In a last attempt to save her they turned to a surgeon who had developed the use of artificial heart pumps for patients with heart failure.

Soon after midnight she was transferred to Oxford. Professor Steven Westaby acted quickly to implant a small battery-powered centrifugal pump into the base of her heart. About the size of an orange and with the appearance of a miniature aeroplane engine, the pump's spinning turbine took over the function of her own failing heart.

The operation worked. The pump was removed 1 week later and the woman's own heart took back the task of keeping her alive. Twelve years later she is a healthy woman with a normal heart.

Professor Westaby has been pioneering the use of heart pumps in Oxford since the mid-1990s, when I was the Chief Executive of the Oxford Radcliffe Hospital, where he worked. His most successful patient to date has lived for 7 years with a pump in his heart, a pack of batteries strapped to his waist and a battery charger close to hand. Some of these devices had been used to keep patients alive whilst they waited for a transplant; but this was the first time that one had been used in this way in the UK as an interim 'bridge' to recovery.

Professor Westaby noticed that some of the hearts taken out of patients when they finally received their transplants showed signs of recovery. Resting them, whilst the pump did the work, seemed to help them to recover some of their old resilience and muscular strength. Perhaps, he wondered, blood pumps might have a wider role in helping hearts to recover. He has subsequently set up a research programme to try to understand more about what is happening within the metabolism of the heart muscle and what role genetics may play.

This is a story made for journalism or the big screen and is a wonderful example of what modern medicine can do. It shows off the skill of doctors and other clinical staff, describes pioneering methods and illustrates very effectively the link between conventional surgery, new technology and genetics. It shows us that medicine and healthcare are still improving and allows us to believe that, given enough resources, even the most impossible sounding challenges may yet be met.

It is not the whole story however. This chapter describes some of the great successes of the last century but also shows how some very deep-seated problems have developed alongside them over the years. Many, perhaps most people, recognize these problems and many people working in health have ideas about how they should be solved. We are not short of analysis or prescription. The problem is implementation – how to make the changes that are necessary.

The three levels for action on health

We have experienced extraordinary improvements in health in the UK and other western countries over the last century. In the last chapter I described how poorer countries needed a combination of improvements in health services, measures to tackle poverty and social change if they were going to improve their health. We can use the same analysis here to show how richer countries have benefited from just such a combination of action on health, action on poverty and social change.

If we take the UK as an example, life expectancy at birth has risen by 30 years over the last century and quality of life has changed dramatically. There are more and better treatments for our many ailments and we can have our hips replaced, our cataracts removed and our arteries re-vascularized as a matter of routine. Roads and workplaces are far safer, housing and drains are better, and smoking is, at last, reducing. Health promotion and healthcare have added years to life and life to years.

It would be difficult to overstate these changes. When the Royal College of Obstetrics and Gynaecology was founded in 1929 a mother in the UK had about a 1 in 250 chance of dying with each child born,[1,2] similar to the current figures for Sudan or India.[3] Her great granddaughter's risk now is about 1 in 15 000.[4]

We are now mostly more affluent, fitter and healthier and have easier and more comfortable lives than our parents and grandparents. There is still poverty today although its impact is, in absolute terms at least, far less extreme. Before the National Assistance Acts of 1911 and 1946 and the establishment of the National Health Service in 1948, many people couldn't afford any kind of healthcare and the illness or disability of a breadwinner was often catastrophic for a family, just as it is today in so many poor countries.

Social change has also been profound with far greater access to education, much better employment conditions and a range of benefits available to people to provide for disability, old age and unemployment. When the retirement age for men in the UK was set at 65 in 1925, pensioners only expected a few more years of life at most. Today, less than a century later, we can expect a healthy 'third age' to take us up to and into our 80s.

Figure 3.1, which is by no means comprehensive, illustrates some of the different actions that between them have contributed in some way to health. I have chosen to mention some that are legislative, some purely medical and some that are the result of popular campaigns or private sector or individual action. This, too, reflects the way that health improvement will come in poorer countries with the involvement of the public, not-for-profit and private sectors and civil society.

These events listed here do not make up a coherent whole nor are they all linked together in any direct way. Indeed, some may have moved the country in opposite

	Health	**Wealth**	**Social change**
1976–2008	Genome decoded Control of tobacco Keyhole surgery New drug development Some cancers alleviated Hip, knees and cataracts surgical replacements Seatbelt and drink driving legislation	Minimum wage Childhood poverty programmes Equal pay legislation De-regulation of employment	Rapid expansion of use of information and communications technology into social networking and elsewhere Sure start and nursery education Expansion of universities Anti-discrimination legislation Rise in school leaving age
1951–1975	Open heart surgery Clean Air Act 1956 to reduce air pollution	Rising standards of living and availability of consumer goods and technology	Health and Safety legislation Contraception and family planning Expansion of universities and Education Act 1962 – university students' grant scheme
1926–1950	Creation of the welfare state with the launch of the National Health Service in 1948, the 1944 Education Act creating free universal secondary education, the 1945 Family Allowance Act, the 1946 National Insurance Act, the 1948 National Assistance Act and the 1948 Children Act		
	Penicillin (1928) and the start of modern antibiotics	Development of campaigns for better working conditions and equal pay for women	Votes for women
1900–1925	Safer anaesthetics (intravenous) 1920 Improved medical education, expansion of the medical Royal Colleges	1911 National Insurance Act covering health and unemployment First old-age pensions introduced in 1908	1906 Education Act offering free school meals and the School Medical Service

Figure 3.1 The three levels for action on health – applied to the UK (1900–2008)

directions from others. Some are the result of a particular political project or movement, but some aren't. Perhaps controversially, I have suggested here that both the earlier campaigns for better working conditions and the later de-regulation of employment contributed in their time to reducing poverty and therefore improving health.

Readers will undoubtedly identify different candidates for inclusion here and feel that I have left out key players and key events. I have. The purpose is to illustrate in very broad terms one country's route to health improvement. It paints a picture of a population that is becoming richer, whose education and quality of life are improving and which is living longer and more healthily. It illustrates the potential for linkages between better education, improved standards of living and the promotion of health and healthy behaviours. Crucially, we need to remember that the route to further health improvement will involve all these three areas of health, wealth and social change.

A figure like this for a Scandinavian country would contain even more social and economic legislation and regulation; one for the USA would contain far less public activity and far more private enterprise. The Scandinavians have created a more equal society with higher average life expectancy, the Americans one with greater inequalities in everything including life expectancy, where the average is lower. There is no single route to take and countries will live with the consequences good and bad of the one they choose.

The most influential series of events in social policy in the twentieth century was the publication of the Beveridge report in 1942 and the subsequent creation of the welfare state in the middle and late 1940s, where the establishment of the NHS was accompanied by the reform and expansion of social security assistance and education. We are living with the consequences, good and bad, today and any political and social reformer needs to take account of them.

Equally, we are living with the history described in the 'health' column where the Royal Colleges and other institutions consolidated their power in the early part of the century, negotiated a central position for themselves in the new NHS in 1948 and are now part of an explosion of invention and activity in the last quarter-century. This history has brought great benefits, but it has also bred its own problems.

The woman from Reading

There are many good reasons to expect this remarkable progress in rich countries to carry on with continuing improvements in all three areas. Populations are getting wealthier and becoming better educated, scientific discovery continues and clinical expertise, aided by new technologies, is constantly improving. Professor Westaby and his colleagues will be able to do even more remarkable things in the future.

However, all is not well even today and we can hear many stories about patients' experiences that are very different to the experience of the young woman in Oxford. Just as the UK 'health, wealth and social change' figure mirrors events in other countries, these stories can be found in any country with a developed western-style health system.

As Chief Executive of the NHS I saw some of the very best of the NHS, where people received extraordinary treatment and excellent care. I also saw some of the worst complaints from patients and met some of the people worst affected by poor-quality treatment. Reading those accounts and meeting these people were depressing and salutary experiences.

Shocked by one such case, I asked each Chief Executive and Chair of an NHS hospital, health authority and primary care organisation personally to shadow a patient who had a chronic disease and to discuss what they had learned with their Board at the next meeting. I wanted all of us to gain a better understanding of what it was like to have a long-term condition and to need to keep coming back to the NHS for care and treatment. I did the same myself and spent time with a woman in Reading who had experienced a whole series of health problems over 30 years. She suffered or had suffered from many different ailments and had been investigated, operated on and cared for by many different NHS organisations.

I sat in her front room and listened with amazement as she and her husband, now her full-time carer, told me stories about her cancers, her heart attack, the time she was in renal failure and no one had realised and the different time when a quick-thinking doctor had saved her life. Now she needed long-term care for a number of conditions and used some NHS services every week.

She, like Professor Westaby's patient, was an exception and few other people can have had her range of experiences, both good and bad. Her experience did, however, throw light on what it was like to be a patient with some of the more common problems that the NHS has to deal with on a regular basis. She was different simply because she had had a lot of them and had therefore tested the system out pretty thoroughly. She was very grateful for all the help she had received but told me, ticking them off on her hands as she spoke, that there were four things we could definitely do better.

The first thing was that she wanted whichever health professional she was seeing at any given time to be aware of all her health problems and to be able to talk with her about them all and help coordinate her care. She knew very well that she would need different specialists for her heart and her diabetes, but she did want to know how the different treatments related and, at the most practical level, that her hospital and family practitioner appointments would be coordinated wherever possible.

She also wanted, in the word of Don Berwick, the leading expert on quality improvement and founder of the Institute for Healthcare Improvement, to know that the system remembered her and knew who she was.

Warming to the task, she went on to describe to me, secondly, how badly referrals from one NHS organisation to another were sometimes managed and how, even within an organisation, the different departments were frequently not good at communicating with each other. Her experiences echoed what other people had told me. It also reminded me that some people had even worse problems. Users of mental health services, in particular, often have great difficulty in receiving physical care, whilst patients with physical illnesses frequently find it very hard to obtain mental health treatment.

Her third complaint was also one I had heard before: "Something almost always goes wrong". She had endured major problems with the service on a few occasions, but found that minor problems occurred on almost every occasion. This was almost always true of her times in hospital where there may be 100 or more interactions between staff and patients in an average stay, covering everything from mealtimes to drug rounds and from diagnosis to treatment. There was a lot to go wrong and something almost always did. Some of these problems appeared to her to be important, like the name of a medicine spelled wrongly or an x-ray missing; most were irritating problems like being kept waiting, being given contradictory information about an appointment or not having messages passed on to her.

A study in the USA showed that 55% of these staff–patient interactions are carried out fully satisfactorily with the patient receiving the appropriate scientifically indicated care. In other words, in every case approaching half of the things done or not done to a patient are inappropriate in some minor or, occasionally, major way. The authors' conclusion was that: "The 'Defect Rate' in the technical quality of American health care is approximately 45%."[5] There is no reason to think it would be particularly different in other rich countries.

Her final complaint was about communication and about whether people listened to her or kept her informed. She gave me several examples where, if someone had explained things better or more fully, she would have been able to head off problems herself. "And, of course", she pointed out to me, "things would have gone better if they had listened to me". This may or may not always have been true, but she certainly knew a lot about her own problems and her treatments.

None of these problems are unique to the UK. Reviews of patients' experiences and their complaints from around the world reveal very similar patterns, with some countries scoring better on some aspects and worse on others. The Commonwealth Fund, which conducted a review of patients' reported experiences in six of the richest countries in the world, looked at, among other things, whether patients felt that they had been given a good enough explanation of their condition and treatment. No country received better than a 66% good rating. The UK was in the middle.[6]

These two stories, from Oxford and Reading, come from my own personal experience and observation but it would be very easy to replicate them from other observers and from other countries. They illustrate how health services are better at dealing with some sorts of patients than others and that typically, it is patients with multiple conditions and more complex needs who miss out.

The NHS is an integrated system with everyone working to the same basic procedures and protocols, yet even we didn't get it right. Countries with large numbers of independent providers, each of which may well focus on their particular role and boundaries, have a more difficult problem. A patient visiting different hospitals or physicians may receive very different care in the different places, may have no way of joining them up and, as a result, their care may be poorer and the risk of something going wrong may be higher.

The woman from Reading raised profound issues about the way the NHS operated in practice. She was in effect telling me that her care wasn't well coordinated, that different clinicians and services didn't talk to each other, there were too many little mistakes made as well as some big ones and that health workers neither explained things to her clearly nor listened to her thoughts and observations. It was a pretty devastating account even if, as she told me, these things didn't happen all the time and, she said, sweetening the pill, she had experienced wonderful care most of the time.

The NHS Chairs and Chief Executives

The Chairs and Chief Executives also had other things to think about. Top of the list for most of them was the rising expenditure and anxiety that services couldn't be sustained in the future, let alone improved. There was a good basis for this fear. All these new treatments and technologies are expensive, aging populations need more care and the public's expectations of good health and good services continue to rise and they become more demanding.

At the global level we can see these pressures reflected in a very well-established trend across countries whereby as each gets richer it spends a higher proportion of its income on health. Although there is variation between countries, a rough average is that every 1% growth in GDP is accompanied by 1.1% growth in health expenditure. Health costs are eating up more and more of our national wealth and it is not clear how long this trend can be sustained.[7] High-income countries spend on average 9% of their GDP on health, with the USA now spending 16% and rising.[8]

The public recognizes these problems and now, in almost all high-income countries, see health as one of their top worries, alongside the economy and security. Their concern is reflected in the way politicians, President Obama most recently, have given healthcare reform such priority. Speaking to the American Medical Association in June 2009 he said that "Reform is not a luxury, it is a necessity", and went on to say dramatically that "If we do not fix our healthcare system the US may go the way of General Motors – paying more, getting less and going broke."[9]

Whilst President Obama may have been speaking about the costs of health services, it is worth noting that ill health is an enormous cost to the whole economy. It is estimated that ill health costs the UK economy about £100 billion a year in lost production, benefits and taxes, a figure equivalent to the entire UK health budget.[10]

The Chairs and Chief Executives would also have been worried about clinical outcomes and standards and about making sure that their hospital or service was using evidence and best practice in caring for their patients and was not failing them or, worse, damaging the people in their care. They would have known that there is enormous variation in standards of care and in its cost.

The Dartmouth Institute has over the last 20 years documented these variations in the USA, describing in many articles how some hospitals and some States spend twice as much as others, yet achieve the same or lower levels of quality. In a commentary on a recent study, an article in the *New England Journal of Medicine* read: "Patients in high-cost regions have access to the same technology as those in low-cost regions, and those in low-cost regions are not deprived of needed care. On the contrary, the researchers note that care is often better in low-cost areas." The authors argue that "the differences in growth are largely due to discretionary decisions by physicians that are influenced by the local availability of hospital beds, imaging centers and other resources – and a payment system that rewards growth and higher utilization."[11]

In these few words, the commentary exposes problems of variation in quality, waste of resources and a system and professionals driven by what appear to be very perverse incentives. These are fundamental problems.

The Chairs and Chief Executives would also have been aware that even in the NHS, founded on the ideal of equality of access to care, the poorer get a poorer deal. There is growing inequality in health and in health care. We are all becoming fitter, consuming more health care and living longer but the richer are doing this faster than the poor and the differences in health and life expectancy are growing.[12]

The findings of the Commission on the Social Determinants of Health, discussed in the last chapter has relevance in these countries as well as in those with low and middle incomes. The inverse care law, whereby those most in need within any population get least and those least in need get most, applies everywhere.

An observer may feel that most of these problems are simply management and leadership problems and that the Chairs and Chief Executives themselves need simply to do better or to make way for others who can do so. These are of course in part, at least, leadership and management problems. Some systems and some countries do better on these issues than others; however, all struggle.

Why is it so difficult in the UK to provide a joined-up service to the woman from Reading whilst containing costs, offering evidence-based care and making sure it is available to everyone? Why does some care cost twice as much as others in the USA and may be of poorer quality?

At the heart of the problem, I believe, lie three issues that concern management and leadership but also take us into the realms of politics, social and economic structures and values.

Three simple headlines

As with health in poor countries, there are three very simple headlines. The first is that the nature of the diseases we suffer from is changing. The major health problems of the early twenty-first century are not the same as those in the early and middle parts of the twentieth century, when our healthcare systems were formed.

As our populations get older and richer they suffer more from non-communicable diseases such as diabetes, cancer, coronary and vascular disease, all of which are linked to behaviour, diet and lifestyle. These now account for the vast majority of our illness and our health care costs. At the same time we have become much more vulnerable to global pandemics and diseases and to shared health risks such as climate change.

The second headline is that we need new approaches and new services to deal with the new needs of the twenty-first century. Success in avoiding these risks or treating these diseases depends as much on our actions as individuals and as societies as it does on new drugs and technologies, although both are vitally important.

The third headline is very simply that all the incentives of the current system are geared towards maintaining the status quo and keeping things as they are. They are proving a very powerful and resistant barrier to creating new approaches and new services.

To put it at its simplest, the current system can't deal with the new problems and is actually getting in the way of our doing so. The very things that helped us make such excellent progress in the twentieth century have, paradoxically, now become a major part of the problem.

The first headline: the changing pattern of disease in the twenty-first century

The first two headlines, that the diseases we have to deal with have changed and that we need new approaches and services, are relatively straightforward and non-controversial and will be described fairly briefly here. The third headline, that the current system can't deal with the problems and is actually getting in the way, is much more contentious and will be dealt with at greater length.

Life has moved on. Looking back over the last century it is easy to see the changes in the patterns of deaths and illness. Many infectious diseases have been brought under control, deaths of mothers and newborn children have been dramatically reduced, antibiotics have contained infection and there are far fewer industrial injuries and diseases than there were.

Causes of death have changed over the last century: where infectious diseases once dominated, cancer and heart disease now overshadow all other causes. Figure 3.2, which compares causes of death in the UK in 1880 and 1997, illustrates the changes.

The biggest group in 1880 is 'other diseases', which includes many deaths where the causes were ill-defined, non-symptomatic or classified as being caused by old age, and reflects the state of knowledge and administrative systems at the time. Infectious diseases account for 33% of the deaths in 1880, but have fallen 17% in 1997. TB deaths alone fell from 80 000 to 440. By 1997 cancers and circulatory disease accounted for 69% of deaths, where before they were relatively rare or went undetected and amounted to only 10% of deaths.

These are very big changes and have demanded very big changes in services. The biggest impact on health services, however, has been the growth of long-term conditions, where patients require long-term care and which give rise to long-term costs. Cancers and

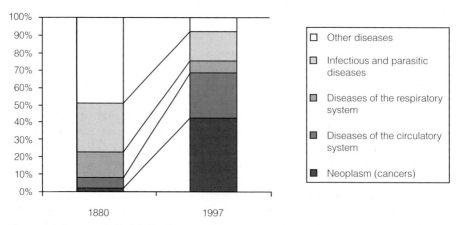

Figure 3.2 Causes of death in England and Wales 1880–1997. From Hicks J, Allen G. *A Century of Change: Trends in UK statistics since 1900.* Social and general statistics section, House of Commons Library. Research paper 99/111. 1999. Available at: www.parliament.uk/commons/lib/research/rp99/rp99-111.pdf

heart and vascular disease may be the ultimate cause of death, but where they once killed swiftly, they are now managed over many years as chronic or long-term conditions. At the same time we have seen a big rise in other long-term conditions, often associated with age, such as diabetes, arthritis and dementia, which may not themselves kill people, but which require care and attention over years.

There has also been a significant increase in long-term mental health problems, partly due to better diagnosis. One in 4 of us will experience some degree of mental illness in our life and for some people it will have a major impact on their health in the long term. Mental illness now accounts for about 12% of NHS costs. Greater affluence has not made us less susceptible to mental illness or happier but, rather, appears to have revealed high levels of mental illness and unhappiness.[13,14]

Taken together it is now these groups with long-term illnesses and long-term needs that account for much the greatest part of healthcare expenditure. Other problems haven't totally gone away. People still need emergency care, contract infections and need operations for one-off problems, but these are not the things making the biggest demands on people and resources.

Analysis shows that the sickest 5% of the US population account for 49% of all healthcare expenditure and the sickest 10% account for 64%; whilst half the population use only 3% of the total expenditure.[15] Looking at a similar analysis in the UK, Figure 3.3 shows that 5% of the population use 42% of inpatient beds, 10% use 53%, whilst half the population only use 10%.[16]

The patients who use most of these resources in the UK, the USA and other richer countries are, unsurprisingly, people with longer term conditions, the regular users or 'frequent fliers' of the healthcare system. They can be grouped in different ways by, for example, different diseases, number of conditions or acuity, but the most interesting I have seen groups them by the combination of factors shown in Figure 3.4.

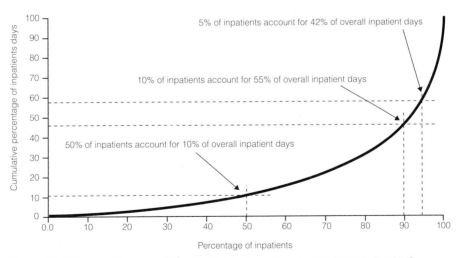

Figure 3.3 UK population usage of inpatient beds. From Department of Health. The NHS Improvement Plan: putting people at the heart of public services. 2004. Available at: www.dh.gov. uk/prod_consum_dh/groups/dh_digitalassets/@dh/@en/documents/digitalasset/dh_4084522.pdf

Group	% of costs
Healthy	6.5
Maternal and infant health	3
Acutely ill, mostly curable	15
Chronic condition, normal function	40
Stable, significant disability	14.5
Short period of decline near death	2.5
Organ system failure	5
Long, dwindling course	13

Figure 3.4 US healthcare percentage of costs for different groups in the population. From Lynn J, Straube B, Bell KM, Jenks SF, Kambic RT. Using Population Segmentation to Provide Better Health Care for All: The 'Bridges to Health' Model. *Milbank Quarterly* 2007; 85: 185–208

The final part of the new mix of diseases and conditions that health systems have to deal with, is, of course, the new infections and diseases, the genuinely new and those like multiple drug-resistant TB that mutated from old ones, which can sweep around the world so easily.

It is worth noting in passing just how different, with the exception of these global problems, the issues faced in rich countries are from those in many poorer ones. However, these non-communicable and long-term problems are starting to appear there and, as we have seen from the last chapter, are already a major problem in South Asia and are giving Africa a double burden of disease. At the same time, with the movement of populations from poorer to richer countries, there has been some changes in disease patterns locally. In London, for example, many of the people with communicable diseases are found amongst these groups.

The second headline: we need new approaches and new services

These new diseases and threats require different approaches and different solutions. We need new services but we also need a much greater emphasis on prevention and health education, getting in early to stop the incipient problems of alcoholism and obesity before and as they start. As the demand changes, the supply side also needs to change.

At the risk of oversimplification, the normal model of hospital care for the last century has been an episodic and linear one. A patient is referred by their GP to a specialist for treatment, they have outpatient appointments and diagnostic tests, are treated in hospital or elsewhere and their problem is dealt with, whether successfully or not.

This, very crudely, resembles a production line where the healthcare system produces a product, in this case an operation or a treatment. The patient is carried along by the flow from one point to the next with relatively little discretion or choice. There may be diversions off the main route for a series of diagnostic tests or further consultations with other specialists but the general structure of the process looks like that in Figure 3.5.

Whilst not all patients are actually handled in this way, the important point here is that this is how the system has been conceived and set up and, crucially, what people are paid

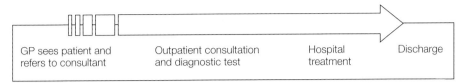

Figure 3.5 The production line

for. Even family practitioners and the UK's General Practitioners practise quite largely in this way with episodic interventions; although they are increasingly adopting more innovative models. In the UK, for example, hospitals are paid for 'episodes of care' and American and other insurance companies largely pay for services on this model. To some extent it is these payments systems that determine the model of care.

It is easy to see how anyone whose needs don't fit this pattern, perhaps because, like the woman from Reading, they have more than one disease or need a mix of care from different people, is going to have problems. Their carers have to bend the system and probably the rules to provide care. It is no wonder it so often goes wrong.

I have heard complaints from doctors and managers in both the UK and the USA that 'the system' doesn't allow them to give the best treatment or, if they do, they don't get paid for it. This is generally the sort of problem they are encountering. Administrative and payment systems reinforce the production line approach. In the UK I have heard doctors complain that they can't set up a diabetic service in the community, where they think it would be better sited than in a hospital, because they can only get paid through the hospital.

In the USA I have listened to a former medical director of the Johns Hopkins Hospital, one of the largest and most prestigious in the country, complaining that he couldn't set up a service the way that was best for his patients because legislation dating from 1964 specified what he could be reimbursed for and what it was legal for him to do. The largely private sector healthcare industry of the USA has, perhaps surprisingly, more regulation in this area than state systems like the NHS.

In practice humane nurses, doctors and managers very often find ways round these restrictions and get things done, despite the system. These problems do, however, illustrate why so many of them are so critical of administration and the administrators bound by the system.

A more appropriate model of care for patients with long-term problems would look something like the 'life belt' illustrated in Figure 3.6, where the patient, at the centre, is able to receive services from any of these sources in turn, in any order. Our health systems need to be able to deliver services based on this sort of model as well as on the episodic 'production line' one – both are needed – and doctors and hospitals need to be able to be paid to do so.

There is now a great deal of understanding and a strengthening consensus amongst health planners and policymakers in richer countries about what needs to be done. Services need to be developed to meet the differing needs of the differing groups of patients; much more attention must be given to patients with long-term conditions and multiple needs, and incentives and systems need to be designed to support these changes.

Underlying all these changes is the recognition that in the twenty-first century, the most significant diseases and problems we are facing relate to our behaviours and our

The Life Belt

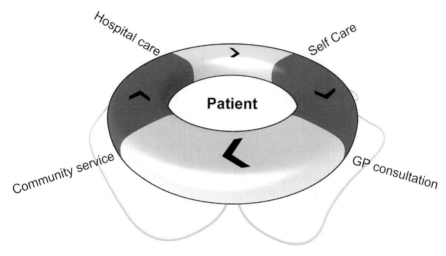

Figure 3.6 The life belt

society, whether we are talking about smoking, alcohol consumption, sexual behaviour or diet. To oversimplify for greater effect: where we once faced diseases that were simply parasitic on our physical bodies, we now face diseases that are also parasitic on our behaviours and on our society.

We need far more effective ways to engage both society and individuals in improving health. The models that are now being developed are generally built on an expectation that patients will play a far more significant role in the future. They are expected to have choices and play an active role in their own care. This is not totally new, of course, the average person with diabetes, after all, provides about 200 hours of self-care in which they medicate, inject and test themselves, for every 2 hours they receive from a professional.

As importantly, family and other carers are now beginning, but only beginning, to be recognized for what they do. They are the biggest support for patients and Carers UK, the national body, estimates that there about 6 million carers in the UK, each of whom does work to the value of more than £15 000 or about £87 billion in total. The NHS now provides support through Carers Direct and private companies are active in supplying home nurses and developing new products for this market.[17]

In the UK and other countries there has also been a great deal of innovation in re-designing services to meet the needs of specific groups of patients. 'Case managers', often nurses, have been employed to guide and look after a patient throughout the system. Navigation aids have been provided for patients faced with daunting choices and apparent confusion. Effort has gone into designing 'patient pathways' so that patients travel through the system in ways that are appropriate to their condition – and, also importantly, are able to see what is happening to them.[16]

David Lawrence, the very experienced former Chairman and CEO of the Kaiser Foundation Health Plan in the USA, writes of the need for a 'balanced health care system' and has identified six core capabilities that are needed by a health system, as shown in Figure 3.7.

At the same time planners, policymakers, academics and business people have been trying to devise ways of ensuring that payment systems reinforce these models and don't undermine them. Service deliverers need to get paid for what they do. In England we radically re-designed the NHS system so that, amongst other things, NHS and other providers had more freedom to innovate and, crucially, that the financial arrangements promoted services designed around patients' needs or, as we put it more colloquially, where 'money followed the patient'.[16]

In the very different environment of the USA, Clayton Christensen, from Harvard Business School, has collaborated with two doctors to apply his model of 'disruptive innovation' to promote an equally radical change in the system. He has treated healthcare in the same way that he would any other industry, promoting the use of technology to simplify processes and developing appropriate business models and the right commercial environment.[18] We can expect to see many new technologies that help monitor progress and support healthcare to be developed over the next few years. They will be accompanied by new business models that utilise the minimal costs of IT and communication to reduce cost and increase coverage.

He shows that, in principle at least, it would be possible to create a high-quality and lower cost system that offers people the services they need. It is a powerful work that offers many insights by treating health as a private sector enterprise subject to all the normal give and take of the market. As such, it explicitly treats health as a commodity, doesn't attempt to deal with the wider social aspects of health and the links with poverty and social structure that we discussed in the last chapter; nor does it take full account of the roles and power of health professionals.

- *Prevention and wellness care to help populations and individuals avoid or minimise illness and make healthy lifestyle choices*

- *Urgent care for people with self-limiting conditions*

- *Chronic disease management*

- *Acute care that is technology intensive*

- *Navigation support to help individuals choose*

- *Cure-to-palliation support*

Figure 3.7 The six core capabilities needed by different groups of patients. From Lawrence D. Presentation at Inaugural meeting of the Forum for Personal Health. Seattle, Washington, 18 June 2009

If the problems are so well understood and all this brainpower has been applied to them, why, we may ask, is it proving so difficult to tackle them? Why can't we just change the service and business models? Why can't we have 'life belts' as well as 'production lines'? Why can't we change the system?

This takes us on to the third simple headline in which I asserted that the current system itself was a major obstacle to progress.

The third headline: the power of the system

The problems here are twofold. Firstly, so many institutions and so many people from the health professions, science, commerce and government have so much invested in the current system, and therefore have so much to lose by change. Secondly, the public, politicians and patients are almost all conditioned by history to think about health and healthcare in particular ways. It is for these reasons that we are not just dealing with leadership and management problems but need to address political, economic and social issues.

It should be stressed at the outset of this discussion, of course, that we are indebted to many of these institutions and individuals, singly and in combination, for so much progress over the last century and longer. It is the very lack of them in poorer countries, as we saw in the last chapter, which means so many people suffer and die. However, their very success, translated into power and influence, is now causing problems.

Before looking at this in greater detail we need to sidetrack briefly to consider a very important distinction between public or population health on the one hand and clinical medicine on the other. It is worth spending a moment on this here as it helps explain the problem and point the way towards solutions.

I am using 'public health' here in the British tradition to mean everything that affects the health of the public or the population in an area or country. It includes such things as the provision of clean air and water, good nutrition and safe roads. It seeks to improve the health of the whole population, whilst clinical professionals give care and treatment to their individual patients.

The story of how public health has developed in the UK has many similarities with the situation in poorer countries today. Many of the great gains of the nineteenth and early twentieth century were due to matters as seemingly simple as clean water, safer working environments and public education.

It is a story of scientific observation and research from the time of John Snow in the mid-nineteenth century, who memorably identified a water pump in Clapham as the source of a cholera outbreak and shut it down, to the work of current researchers on topics as diverse as the impacts of climate change or of family structures.[19] Engineering and technology have also played their part. The nineteenth century engineer Sir Joseph Bazalgette built the sewers of London and thereby eliminated the 'great stink' arising from the open sewer of the Thames, with all its accompanying diseases.[20] Modern-day engineers tackle pollution and ensure we have clean air and safe working environments.

Florence Nightingale was a public health pioneer who used her remarkable mathematical ability to analyse deaths in the Crimea and realise that infection was a greater killer than battle. In later life she was very conscious of the impact of 'poisonous air' and wanted her new hospital built in the fresh air of the countryside and far from the dangerous banks of the Thames. On what must have been a very rare occasion for this remarkable and remarkably persistent reformer, she didn't get her way and the new development of St Thomas's was built facing Parliament across the river in the heart of London.[21]

It is also a story of public campaigns and public education. Today we are very familiar with all the efforts to stop us from smoking and to encourage us to eat healthily, exercise and have safe sex lives. Looking back on earlier generations in the UK we can see that there were campaigns for people to register with the family doctors available through the new National Health Service and for mass screening for TB and a very strong emphasis on teaching girls about health and how to look after their families. All of these would seem very familiar to a public health worker in Africa or India today.

Public health can lay claim to creating the foundation for all the improvement in health we have seen over the last century or longer. Its impact has been profound. Looking forward, the discipline has much more to offer. Analysis from the WHO shows that all the most cost-effective health interventions are public health rather than clinical ones. They are about immunisation, clean water and the education of girls in poorer countries and about lifestyle changes in richer ones.[22]

Despite both the successes of the past and its potential for the future, public health has become, in effect, the junior partner to clinical medicine and been less powerful and less well funded. On the surface this appears to be largely accidental or due to decisions taken explicitly or implicitly in different countries at the beginning of the last century to separate the two disciplines and train people differently for each. Underlying this is a story of money and power.

Medicine has ancient roots, going back thousands of years with the western scientific tradition starting in the last 500 years as universities became more active in medicine and the first standard setting body, the Royal College of Physicians, being established in London in 1518. It was only in the nineteenth century and beginning of the twentieth, however, that the practice of clinical medicine was at last put onto a regulated and unassailable scientific basis thanks to the Medical Act of 1858 in the UK and the work of pioneers such as Abraham Flexner in 1910 in the USA. Previously 'quacks' of all types flourished in a society that permitted 'doctors' to practise largely at will.[23]

These European and American developments have been hugely influential internationally and helped ensure the development of western scientific medicine as a distinctive body of knowledge and practice throughout the world. Over the past century it has become the dominant model globally, carried around the world with colonisation and trade. It has, as we shall see, allied itself with scientific research and commerce and secured the backing and funding of governments.[24]

At around the same time, the discipline of public health, which has its own long and distinguished history, became largely separated from clinical medicine. In the USA the Rockefeller Foundation's Welch-Rose Report of 1915 set barriers between the two that last to this day and, whilst the separation was less rigid in the UK and Europe, clinical medicine has continually become more powerful and influential, eclipsing its near relative.[25]

Public health has over the years had revivals and reinvented itself, experiencing brief periods when its importance was recognised. It has never quite managed, however, to link itself sufficiently closely to the scientific establishment and commercial interests to challenge the hegemony of clinical medicine. Now, with the emergence of global health as a new discipline it is once again being viewed as of enormous importance.

Clinical medicine meanwhile has gone from strength to strength. Its great institutions, its Royal Colleges and Medical Associations, have become very grand and powerful. They have influenced the way populations think about health and largely determined the shape of health services and the whole health industry. Flexner and others not only sorted out the quacks from the professionals, they consolidated the power of the clinical medical profession.

The last century has seen science and medicine advancing together as a few simple examples remind us. The first antibiotics ended the grip of pneumonia, the 'old man's friend' and a major cause of postoperative mortality, in the 1940s. Churchill, whilst Prime Minister and at war with Germany, was successfully treated for pneumonia with the new drug M and B in 1940 in what seems to be a clear case of science changing the course of history or, perhaps more accurately, making sure that it didn't change.

More recently the pharmacological and technological advances in anaesthesia have meant that a consultant retiring after a 40-year career today has seen spectacular changes in how much control the new drugs and equipment give them and seen the risk of a patient succumbing under anaesthetic reducing to less than 1 in 250 000.[26]

Medical imaging has developed enormously with scanners using x-rays, magnetic resonance and sound waves able to assist diagnosis and reduce the need for investigative surgery or for time-consuming biological and chemical tests. As their capability grows scientists and clinicians are able to discover more and more about how our bodies work and interact with the environment. Functional MRI scanners now allow us to see what brain activity corresponds with our moods and feelings and offers the promise of better understanding of the physical aspects of mental illness.

Genetics, the development of new computer-controlled and -designed technology and the power of connection and analysis available to every scientist in a rich country drives scientific advance apace. We are entering a world of genetic engineering and personal medicine where we have no idea of the limits to discovery and invention and where all things seem possible.

Commerce and industry have worked alongside the scientists and the professions in the development of new treatments and technologies. Whilst public and private universities and research institutes have undertaken most of the basic research, private enterprise and the search for profit have generally driven the development of the new drugs and therapies, the imaging and the creation of new diagnostic tools. In many other cases it is the commercial businesses that have invested the very large sums needed for development. New drugs have depended on private sector funding, as have many new technologies such as the heart pump used by Professor Westaby in Oxford.

Government is also linked in closely with these other partners of the professions, the scientists and the businessmen. Health is big business. Pharma and health-related technology companies are amongst the largest companies in the world, whilst health insurers and private healthcare companies are a significant and powerful part of some national economies. In Massachusetts, home to a vast medical industry, healthcare represents more than 20% of the economy and pays the wages of more than 1 in 7 of the working population. Bioscience and biomedicine are now the largest contributors to the UK economy, other than the financial services, and the fastest growing of them all.

This economic profile means that health is a significant political and governmental issue and makes for a complicated relationship between business and government. In the UK the Department of Health set up the Pharmaceutical Industry Competitiveness Task Force to support the development of the industry whilst at the same time negotiating reduced prices for the NHS for their products.

This juxtaposition makes explicit something that may be hidden in other countries where the health system is not so directly the responsibility of government. In virtually every rich country, however, government will have an interest both in protecting its industry, whether it is pharmaceuticals or anything else, and in controlling the costs to its population through regulation, subsidy or other means.

Government has proved to be a very generous funder of healthcare as Figure 3.8 shows. In 1920 the Government of the UK spent less than 1% of its GDP on health.[27] By 2005 it was spending about 7% of GDP.[28] The USA spent very little public money on health in the first half of the century and only reached 1% of GDP by 1964. Thereafter, spending accelerated and public expenditure in the USA, too, reached 7% of GDP in 2006.[29,30] Both countries subsidise health to a remarkably similar degree. The big difference between the two countries, of course, is that the USA spends a further 9% of GDP from private sources, mainly insurance, bringing its total to 16%; whilst the UK only spends about 1.5% of private money, bringing its total spend to 8.5% of GDP.

Whilst the private spend on health in the UK is not very high, countries like the USA with a largely private system have also seen a very large increase in private spending. The greater part of this increase has come in the second half of the twentieth century, with growth accelerating particularly steeply in the last quarter.

Both this public policy and these private actions reflect the strong desire of citizens to see more spent on health in order to improve their lives. Politicians and policymakers

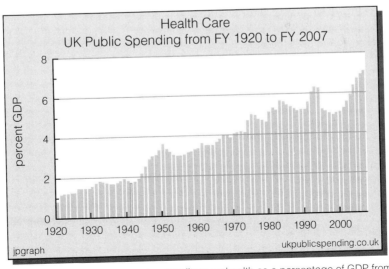

Figure 3.8 UK growth in government expenditure on health as a percentage of GDP from 1920 to 2007. From www.ukpublicspending.co.uk

are responding to public opinion here as well as creating it. Greater wealth has raised the priority richer populations give to health or, to put it another way, greater affluence and leisure have given people more time to worry about the quality of their health and their lives rather than simply struggle for survival.

Different health systems but common assumptions

This account has brought out the close relationship between all the big players in health and healthcare. This has been enormously beneficial and it has also created problems. You don't have to be a conspiracy theorist to see that there is a medico-academic-commercial-governmental alignment of interests that could work to the benefit of patients, but which may not (Figure 3.9).

These powerful linkages have, inevitably, also driven self-interest, created hierarchy and elites and, over time, become self-referring, closed and resistant to change. It has promoted the insider interests of its practitioners, whether they are scientists, doctors, businessmen or government officials, and neglected the changing interests of its beneficiaries, its patients and its customers.

The way the system works reinforces this. The McKinsey Foundation in looking at why the US costs were so much higher than those of any other country concluded that there were two main factors. The first was a far higher rate of investigation and of hospitalization. The second was the almost complete absence of anyone in the system who had an incentive to reduce expenditure. In fact, the Foundation found that hospitals, physicians and suppliers alike had strong incentives to provide more treatment, even if patient benefits were very small or non-existent.[31]

In particular it is the triad of the professions, commerce and technology that has driven costs. Commerce has marketed the products of technology with the active involvement of the professions. All three parties are strongly incentivised to do more, treat more patients and increase overall costs. None are incentivised to manage costs or control waste.

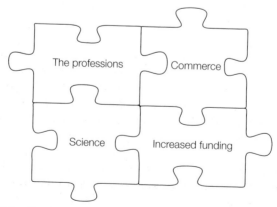

Figure 3.9 Maintaining the status quo – an alignment of interests

We, as the public, are also active participants in this process with our apparent belief that greater expenditure is always a good thing and should always bring greater benefit. This interaction is well illustrated by the account given in the *New York Times* of a doctor being asked by fellow doctors to join them in purchasing the latest CT scanner.

He is tempted and you can understand why. It will be a new service he can offer patients. He will be popular with his colleagues and it will probably be a good investment. Altogether it sounds like a win–win situation. He resists, however, because he is worried that he and the other doctors in the clinic would feel pressure to give scans to people who might not need them in order to pay for the equipment. Yet, the article goes on to say, more than 1000 other cardiologists and hospitals have installed CT scanners on this basis.[32] Not everyone will resist the temptation.

These pressures play out differently in different countries. Countries have their own ways of defining and organizing their role in health and have created very different systems. In very broad terms there are typically European-style systems based on some notion of social solidarity, funded through tax or social insurance, and American-style private systems, funded, in principle at least, through private or employment-based insurance schemes. There are some other very significant variations in how this works in practice. Singapore, for example, has created its own distinctive and successful hybrid, where individuals have their own budgets in part funded by the state but can top them up privately.

For Europeans, again very broadly, the health of individuals and the population as a whole is seen as something of public concern and governments have a proper role in making sure people have access to healthcare and are protected from disease. Health, in economists' terms, is a public good. In the USA, very broadly, people are expected and expecting to look after themselves with the state providing a safety net and protecting the interests of the country as a whole. Health is largely considered a private good, which citizens should seek and provide for themselves in a healthcare marketplace.

In reality, whilst these broad generalisations accurately reflect the prevailing politics and the rhetoric, they gloss over the fact that there is a great deal of similarity in what happens in practice. The social solidarity systems mostly allow people to opt out and 'go private' and to use elements of the different public and private systems at different times, depending on nationally or locally determined rules and procedures. Similarly, the private systems operate safety nets and private philanthropy plays a more substantial role. Moreover, as we have already noted in this chapter, the USA and UK subsidise healthcare to about the same extent.

These differences do matter, however, because whilst American systems, as the McKinsey Foundation report shows, incentivise more activity and treatment, European systems, with resources pooled, will incentivise action to promote the health of whole populations and be more likely to seek cheaper solutions and weigh treatments against each other. If the risk in the private system may be overtreatment or no treatment, the risk in the public system is more likely to be undertreatment. One rations access by cost, the other through explicit decision making.

The differences between the systems appear clearly in the attitudes and opinions of citizens of the different countries. Many Americans are appalled at the thought of what they see as European 'socialised medicine', which would limit their choices over healthcare. Similarly, many Europeans are appalled by what they conceive as a totally private system that gives no attention to the poorest and sickest in the population and where 'the devil takes the hindmost'.

The spectre of 'socialised medicine' is one that opponents of President Obama's healthcare reform are keen to use in the current debates. Michael Moore's film *Sicko* goes in the opposite direction and applauds European systems whilst ridiculing the US system, or lack of it. The differences between the European and American approaches have become a real cause for conflict and, as always with conflict people lose sight of the reality.

These simple examples are rich in cultural and political differences. They serve to show the very different assumptions that people bring to their thinking about health and healthcare and to their approaches to technology. As we shall see in Chapter 5, where I talk about the current race for influence in Africa, these different cultural attitudes also underpin the thinking that informs the different approaches to international development and can lead to unhelpful conflict.

Whilst rich countries make different assumptions about the balance of the role of the state and the individual and about solidarity versus personal responsibility, their institutions and systems nevertheless share a very similar range of assumptions in other areas. These are assumptions about the position and responsibilities of the professions, the importance of science and technology, about governance and accountability, and about the roles ascribed to patients and citizens, and, as important as any of the others, an assumption that greater spending means greater improvement. They are implicit and sometimes explicit in our healthcare systems and institutions.

These assumptions, with only a degree of exaggeration, cast the individual as someone who needs to be educated and persuaded to adopt the right course of action, accepts without question the outcomes of science and research, is a largely passive and patient recipient of care from the professionals, is a consumer who is sold services and who, of course, is paying an increasingly large proportion of their personal income and taxes to support health improvement and, with it, a whole healthcare industry.

Strong professional groups, for example, which led such improvement in the twentieth century, tend to disempower their patients and restrict their ability to make decisions about their own health. Patients who have long-term chronic diseases, like the woman from Reading, often know a great deal about their own health yet can find it very difficult to get doctors and nurses to listen to them. Many people still can't see or own a copy of their own medical record; doctors have to act on their behalf.

It is ironic that many individuals in rich countries, patients and the public, share a sense of powerlessness about their health with people in poor countries. The context is very different in the two cases. People in poor countries need more resources and strengthened health systems. In rich countries, however, the system itself is so strong and so well resourced that it takes the power away from its citizens.

As the public we have played our part in creating this dependence. We have learned to constantly want more from our scientists and professionals. The professions and the professionals have become overmighty and the drug companies overstrong. We have become dependent on ever-growing amounts of money being spent in healthcare and, often, demanded it from our politicians.

These assumptions, which may have seemed unexceptional to many people only 20 or 30 years ago, are now, however, coming under increasing individual and collective

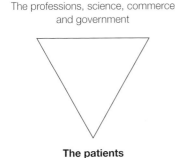

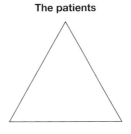

Figure 3.10 Turning the system upside down

scrutiny. It is evident that many people are not satisfied with the roles ascribed to them as patients and consumers of health and they are beginning to break away from the assumptions and biases of the institutions and systems.

Increasingly patients and the public want to see the system turned upside down so that, as Figure 3.10 suggests, the burden and weight of the whole system does not bear down on the patients making them conform, but rather the patients sit above the system drawing on it as they need to. There is plenty of evidence, as I shall show later, that the triangle is turning. Many doctors as well as patients want to see change and are making it happen wherever they can.

Conclusions

The problems described here are enormous and their solutions both difficult and very long term. We need to look in a great deal more detail at what is happening around the world, to understand better some of the social trends that are affecting us all and to learn from the pioneers and innovators, wherever they are to be found.

At this stage we can draw some preliminary conclusions:

- Continuing efforts need to be put into the design of services tailored for different groups of people.
- Administrative systems and business models need to be re-designed to support these services.
- The role of patients and the public in any system need to be strengthened in whatever way fits the culture of the country.
- Public health and clinical medicine need to be brought back closer together, with greater attention and status given to the former.

There are also many outstanding questions, of which the biggest are:

- How can we change the system we have so that it focuses more on public and population health as well as on reducing waste and improving quality?

- How can we possibly make the changes we need against the opposition of all the powerful institutions and forces with vested interests in the status quo, what Michael Birt of the Pacific Health Summit has called the 'legacy push-back'?

We will be looking in future chapters at how we can combine insights from poorer countries about population health with experience from richer countries of systematic ways of making quality improvements in services. We will also be considering how it might be possible to generate the power and energy we need for change. In the meantime it is worth remembering that we are dealing here with the problems of success. The systems we have were developed to deal with one set of problems. Their very success in dealing with them means that the problems have moved on.

Our search for understanding continues in the next chapter by beginning our exploration of the relationships between richer and poorer countries.

References

1. Royal College of Obstetricians and Gynaecologists. *History of the College*. [Online]. Available at: www.rcog.org.uk/about-us.
2. Loudon I. Maternal mortality in the past and its relevance to developing countries today. *Am J Clin Nutr* [Online]. 2000; **72**: 241S–6S. Available at: www.ajcn.org/cgi/reprint/72/1/241S. [Accessed 23 September 2009].
3. World Health Organisation. *Maternal Mortality in 2005*. Report number: WQ 16. Available at: www.who.int/making_pregnancy_safer/documents/9789241596213/en/index.html.
4. *Saving Mothers' Lives: Reviewing maternal deaths to make motherhood safer – 2003–2005*. Confidential enquiry into maternal and child health, 2007. Available at: www.cmace.org.uk/getattachment/927cf18a-735a-47a0-9200-cdea103781c7/Saving-Mothers--Lives-2003-2005_full.aspx.
5. McGlynn E, Asch SM, Adams J et al. The quality of health care delivered to adults in the United States. *N Engl J Med* 2003; **348**: 2635–45.
6. Schoen C, Osborn R, Huynh PT, Doty M, Zapert K, Peugh J, Davis K. *Taking the Pulse of Healthcare Systems Experiences of Patients with Health Problems in Six Countries*. The Commonwealth Fund, 2005. Available at: www.commonwealthfund.org/usr_doc/870_Schoen_pulse_HA_itl.pdf?section=4039.
7. Gottret P, Schieber G. *Health Financing Revisited: A practitioner's guide*. Washington: World Bank, 2006.
8. The Henry J. Kaiser Family Foundation. *The Healthcare Marketplace Project: Health care spending in the United States and OECD countries*, 2007. Available at: www.kff.org/insurance/snapshot/chcm010307oth.cfm.
9. Remarks made by the President at the Annual Conference of the American Medical Association. The White House, June 15, 2009. Available at: www.whitehouse.gov/the_press_office/Remarks-by-the-President-to-the-Annual-Conference-of-the-American-Medical-Association/.
10. Black C. *Working for a Healthier Tomorrow*. Dame Carol Black's Review of the health of Britain's working age population. 2008. Available at: www.workingforhealth.gov.uk/documents/working-for-a-healthier-tomorrow-tagged.pdf.
11. Fisher ES, Skinner JS. Getting past denial – The High Cost of Health Care in the United States Jason M. Sutherland. *N Engl J Med* 2009. Available at: healthcarereform.nejm.org/?p=1739.
12. House of Commons. *Health Committee Report on Health Inequalities*. 2009. Available at: www.publications.parliament.uk/pa/cm200809/cmselect/cmhealth/286/286.pdf.
13. Layard R. *Happiness: Lessons from a new science*. London: Penguin, 2005.
14. Avner O. *The Challenge of Affluence: Self-control and well-being in the United States and Britain since 1950*. Oxford: Oxford University Press, 2006.
15. Zuvekas SH, Cohen JW. Prescription drugs and the changing concentration of Health Care Expenditures. *Health Affairs* 2007; **26**: 248–57.
16. Department of Health. *The NHS Improvement Plan: Putting people at the heart of public services*. 2004. Available at: www.dh.gov.uk/prod_consum_dh/groups/dh_digitalassets/@dh/@en/documents/digitalasset/dh_4084522.pdf.

17. Carers UK. [Press release] 20 September 2007.

18. Christensen CM, Grossman JH, Hwang J. *The Innovator's Prescription: A disruption solution for health-care*. New York: McGraw-Hill, 2009.

19. Vinten-Johansen P, Brody H, Paneth N, Rachman S, Rip M, Zuck D. *Cholera, Chloroform, and the Science of Medicine: A life of John Snow*, New York: OUP, 2003.

20. Halliday S. *The Great Stink of London: Sir Joseph Bazalgette and Cleansing of the Victorian Capital.* Gloucestershire: Sutton Publications, 1999.

21. Nightingale F. Notes on Nursing: What it is and what it is not. New York: D. Appleton and Company, 1859.

22. World Health Organisation. *Primary Health Care: Now more than ever*. The world health report, 2008. Available at: www.who.int/whr/2008/whr08_en.pdf.

23. Beck AH. The Flexner report and the standardization of American medical education. *JAMA* 2004; **291**: 2139–40. Available at: jama.ama-assn.org/cgi/content/full/291/17/2139.

24. Berliner HB. A larger perspective on the Flexner report. *Int J Health Serv* 1975; **5**: 559–74.

25. Fee E. *The Welch-Rose Report: A Public Health Classic.* A publication of the Delta Omega Alpha Chapter to mark the 75th Anniversary of the founding of the John Hopkins University School of Hygiene and Public Health 1916–1992. Available at: www.deltaomega.org/WelchRose.pdf.

26. Royal College of Anaesthetists. *The history of anaesthesia.* [Online]. Available at: www.rcoa.ac.uk/index.asp?PageID=200. [Accessed 23 September 2009].

27. Ukpublicspending.co.uk. Available at: www.ukpublicspending.co.uk/download_ukgs.php?span=ukgs302&year=1920&view=1&expand=&units=p&fy=2009#ukgs302. [Accessed 23 September 2009].

28. World Health Organisation. *United Kingdom.* Available at: www.who.int/countries/gbr/en/. [Accessed 23 September 2009].

29. Usgovernmentspending.com. Available at: www.usgovernmentspending.com/us_health_care_spending_10.html#usgs302. [Accessed 23 September 2009].

30. World Health Organisation. *United States of America.* Available at: www.who.int/countries/usa/en/. [Accessed 23 September 2009].

31. McKinsey Global Institute. *Accounting for the cost of healthcare in the United States.* 2007. Available at: www.mckinsey.com/mgi/rp/healthcare/accounting_cost_healthcare.asp.

32. Berenson A, Abelson R. Weighing the cost of a CT scan's look inside the heart. *The New York Times.* [Online] 29 June 2008. Available at: www.nytimes.com/2008/06/29/business/29scan.html. [Accessed 26 September 2009].

4 Unfair trade (1) – exporting health workers

The facts are plain. Many thousands of health workers who were trained in their own countries have migrated to other countries to work. This is part of a far wider pattern of migration by workers seeking employment and opportunity.[1]

The best estimates are that about 135 000 doctors and nurses who were first trained in Sub-Saharan Africa are now living in richer countries and that many of those graduating in these professions each year will eventually migrate.[2] The position varies enormously from one country to another and from one region of the world to another. However, the underlying pattern is clear: there is now a global labour market in trained health workers and a flow of talent and skill, which goes very largely but not entirely, from poorer countries to richer.

It is equally clear that this export of trained people costs their home countries dearly and that it benefits the richer countries where they now live and work. It is not just countries, of course, that gain and lose from this export and import business. The individuals who leave their own countries mostly gain and those left behind, coping with staff shortages as well as everything else, lose significantly.

Estimates from UN organizations suggest that this export of skilled professionals, not just from the health sector, from Africa costs the continent around US$4 billion a year[3] and that each migrating African professional costs the country about US$184 000.[2] This would mean that the cost of the loss of 135 000 doctors and nurses amounted to over US$24 billion.

This is part of a much greater export of wealth from Africa, where the costs of the wider brain drain across all the educated sectors of society as well as the extraction of natural resources offset the benefits of the flows of inward investment and aid money, some of which, of course, returns to the wealthier country as payment for goods and services.

Richer countries undoubtedly benefit from this migration, whether this is a result of a deliberate policy of undertraining or not. One international recruitment agency estimated in 2008 that the cost of training a doctor in Australia ranges from AU$280 000–400 000, depending on speciality and length of training.[4] The recruitment fee to bring a trained doctor to a job in the country ranges from AU$30 000–60 000. Each migrant doctor could therefore be worth upwards of AU$250 000 in saved costs to the Australian Exchequer. As long ago as 1971 the US Congressional Research Service calculated that the benefit to the US economy from each migrant was about US$20 000 per year.[5]

Although the exact figures can be argued about, we can see that we are dealing with very large sums of money here. These calculations must be pretty compelling if you are only concerned about how to ensure the country has enough doctors and about how to do so within the constraints of you own Australian or American health budget. They are deeply worrying if you are concerned about how to staff your own health service in a poorer country.

The wider story

Whilst this analysis is undoubtedly accurate, it doesn't tell the whole story.

This chapter describes one-half of the unfair import–export business in which poorer countries export, mostly unintentionally and unwillingly, many of their health workers whilst at the same time receiving the, often inappropriate and sometimes discredited, ideas and ideologies of richer countries.

It offers an insight into the many and varied ways in which health workers migrate around the world, with ultimately a net health and economic benefit to richer countries and a net loss to poorer ones. It also describes how emigration together with poor pay and employment practices, bad working conditions, shortfalls in training and lack of resources combine to create a desperate shortage of health workers in many low- and middle-income countries.

The underlying and most significant problem, in terms of numbers, is that not enough health workers are being trained globally, with a particular shortage in low-income countries. Ethiopia, for example, has graduated about 3700 doctors in 20 years, whilst the UK, with a smaller population, now educates almost 8000 a year.[6]

Migration is frequently the subject of a great deal of political attention that sometimes generates more heat than light. The impression is often given that migration is the biggest staffing problem in poorer countries. It isn't. It is important, but the figures show that if every doctor who had migrated were to return to their country of origin it would barely solve 12% of the problem.[7] The 135 000 professionals who have left are only about 8% of Africa's total health workforce, estimated at 1 640 000 in 2006 by the WHO.[8] Many more people need to be trained locally.

The issue of health worker migration is one of the most emotive in healthcare and, as the former Chief Executive of the NHS, I have often been challenged about the UK role in this. Personally, I have no doubt at all that the UK has benefited enormously from waves of health workers coming from the Caribbean, Southeast Asia and Africa and that many of these workers have represented a real loss to their homelands.

I also believe, as I will argue later, that the UK has an obligation to help solve the problem of the lack of health workers in poorer countries. However, my own observations have shown me just how complex this whole field is.

Patterns of migration

The broad patterns of migration over the last 50 years are very clear although, as we shall see later in this chapter, the rise of newly wealthy countries in Asia is bringing new patterns both of emigration and of returning migrants.

There have been large flows of people from former colonies to the former colonial powers where the language, culture and health systems are similar. People have moved from poorer countries to richer ones within their own region with South Africa, for example, benefiting from trained health workers from elsewhere in Africa. The USA has received people from around the world with particularly large numbers from Latin and South America and from India, and with many others coming as 'secondary migrants', after a spell in another country first.

Doctors present much the largest problem in terms of the percentage of people who have emigrated, with in some cases one-third or more of medical students migrating after graduation. More nurses migrate in total, but they represent a much smaller percentage of the numbers trained. The numbers involved are very large as Figure 4.1 shows, with some countries, most notably the UK, the USA, Australia, Canada and New Zealand benefiting from having very large numbers of doctors who had their initial training abroad.

These numbers give us a broad overview of the situation but the world is not a single place and the circumstances and the opportunities as well as the perils facing its citizens are rich and varied. There is a wealth of personal stories and anecdotes, some true and some, perhaps, more fanciful that illustrate this diversity well and present a much more complicated and even confusing picture of migration.

We hear from stories current in the UK, for example, that there is only one paediatrician in Nepal (probably true), there are more Malawian doctors in Manchester than in Malawi (not true, except possibly in some subspecialities) and five times the number of Indian neurosurgeons in the USA than in India (possibly true, but most trained in the speciality in the USA).

We also know, of course, of the migrant who has risen to the top of the profession in their new country, of refugees having the freedom to live and work without constant fear and poverty and of the grandson of a Kenyan goatherder who has become President of the USA.

OECD country	Doctors trained abroad		Nurses trained abroad	
	Number	Percentage of total	Number	Percentage of total
Australia	11 122	21	NA	NA
Canada	13 620	23	19 061	6
Finland	1 003	9	140	0
France	11 269	6	NA	NA
Germany	17 318	6	26 284	3
Ireland	NA	NA	8 758	14
New Zealand	2 832	34	10 616	21
Portugal	1 258	4	NA	NA
United Kingdom	69 813	33	65 000	10
United States	213 331	27	99 456	5

NA, not applicable.

Figure 4.1 Doctors and nurses trained abroad working in OECD countries. From World Health Report 2006 – working together for health. Table 5.1 – doctors and nurses trained abroad working in OECD countries, p98. Available at www.who.int.whr/2006/en/

More prosaically, we know of doctors getting specialist training abroad before returning home, of clinicians sent abroad by their families to earn money and of the governments encouraging emigration because they want the remittances. We also know that temporary migration has brought some benefits, particularly in education and training. The UK and the USA and, to a lesser extent other rich countries, have been and still are the great medical educators of the world. Many people have travelled to these countries for training at all levels, including the most specialist training that they would not have been able to get at home.

Migration is often not a single event in someone's life or, indeed, a once and for all one-way process. Migrants may move from one country to another and on to a third or a fourth. They may acquire new training and skills and they may return home after a few years or retire. Their children may grow up in a foreign country and, at some point in their life return to their parents' country of origin.

Individual examples bring these points to life. The Honourable Socco Kabia became the Health Minister for Sierra Leone in 2008. As a young man he left his country to become a medical student in Germany but returned home as a graduate because he was unable, as a foreigner, to progress on to medical training. He later migrated to the USA for training and worked there for many years.

He returned to Sierra Leone in 2005, following the ending of conflict in his country. Determined to help improve the health of the population, he entered politics and took over one of the most difficult jobs in the world. How does one work to improve health in a population where women have a 1 in 7 lifetime chance of dying in childbirth, 75% of the health workers died in the country's internal conflict or fled the country and you have less than US$5 a year per head of the population to spend on health?

Other Health Ministers in Africa have trained and worked abroad. The Ethiopian Minister has higher degrees from the UK. The Ugandan Minister trained and worked in Chicago for many years as an obstetrician. The last Zambian minister trained and worked as an orthopaedic surgeon in London, UK. There are many other leading doctors in Africa who can tell similar tales.

These personal stories are part of much wider patterns in many countries that go far beyond healthcare. Ben Male fled from his schoolroom in Uganda when Idi Amin's soldiers killed his father. Arriving in Tanzania he was mistaken for a spy by the rebel Ugandans preparing to invade the country and once again had to flee for his life. He was penniless and unable to speak the language when he finally reached safety in Rwanda, where missionaries took him in and cared for the bewildered 17-year-old.

By a remarkable chance the missionaries introduced him to a British schoolteacher who recognized his intelligence and abilities and, raising money from the students at Rugby School, arranged for him to complete his schooling at that archetypal English public school. Ben graduated from Sheffield University and after some years working for NGOs in Europe, returned to Uganda, where he is the country representative for Sightsavers and active in the developing civil society.

Ben is of course an exception both because of his luck and his talent. However, there are many people whose life stories should be recorded both as inspiring in themselves and as being so descriptive of the lives of millions – the lucky and the unlucky – in Africa and in many other poor countries.

Not all migrants are as lucky or as capable as Ben or any of these ministers. Many come to grief on their travels. Unscrupulous traffickers and employers exploit many. Others simply find that their skills are not utilised, their expectations are not met and their hopes are destroyed. London and Washington contain many migrants and refugees whose skills can't be used because of regulations about medical and other practice.

Our existing health institutions tend to behave as if everyone lived the less eventful lives of those in long-settled countries in western Europe. These mobile lives are becoming even more common as borders come down and communication becomes easier. We need to understand this mobility if we are to have a positive impact on managing the damaging effects of migration from poor to rich countries and the effects on the migrants themselves.

On the other side of the equation, people from rich countries choose to work in poorer ones for a whole range of personal reasons. This two-way mobility, with people choosing to work in different countries at different points in their lives, is undoubtedly on the increase.

The success of organizations such as Médecins Sans Frontières, Médecins du Monde, the American Medics, Merlin and others that recruit volunteers to work in poor countries shows just how attractive this lifestyle can be, at least at certain stages in life.

Individuals too have found their own ways to work in their own country and abroad. Chris Lavy worked for many years as a surgeon in Malawi before returning home when his children were at an age when he and his wife wanted them to have English schooling. He is now Professor in the Department of Orthopaedic Surgery at Oxford and manages to combine his work in the UK with continuing involvement in Africa, helping create, for example, the East African College of Surgeons as a means of driving up standards and improving practice.

Philippa Easterbrook, a professor in London, similarly works for long periods in the Infectious Diseases Institute in Kampala. Gordon Williams was Professor of Vascular Surgery at the Hammersmith in London but in 2007 took early retirement to become the first Dean of the St Paul's Millennium Medical School in Addis Ababa. Katrina Percy is one of the youngest executive managers in the NHS. She worked for 2 years in Tanzania as Deputy Director of the Aga Khan Hospital in Dar es Salaam and she is now Chief Executive of Provider Community Services in Hampshire, UK. There are many similar examples across all health disciplines in the UK health sector and many more internationally.

Many middle-aged health professionals from all disciplines and backgrounds, after a career in their own countries, want to do something to help improve health in poorer countries. Even more significantly, very many young people in the UK and the USA see their whole lives differently from older generations and aspire to careers in 'global health'. They are helping to create a new way of looking at the world and their profession, a new global outlook, as will be described in Chapter 9.

These stories raise many questions. They should not take our focus away from the basic fact that the current high levels of export of trained health workers are very damaging to poor countries, but they make us want to explore the reality in more detail in order to understand it better and learn how it might be possible to find some way to reduce or eliminate the damage and, as I will argue, get a fairer price for the export of all this valuable human capital.

Why people migrate

There are many reasons why people migrate; some are directly related to health services, some are not. There are many factors 'pushing' people to leave their own country: from the fear of persecution and the lack of personal and economic security to the sheer frustration of working in awful conditions with no drugs and no equipment and no hope. A survey carried out in the four African countries of Cameroon, South Africa, Uganda and Zimbabwe showed that the four main reasons people emigrated were to achieve better remuneration, a safer environment, better living conditions and better facilities.[8]

Discussions with people in the International Council of Nurses revealed that their feedback from nurses told them that the main reason that nurses emigrate or leave the profession in poor countries are the working environment and the facts that they can't get adequate housing, access to services or schools for their children.

Families also influence the decision to leave. In many parts of the world a university graduate is expected to earn a high income both to benefit themselves and for their, often very extended, families. Many of these families understand very well that there is much more money to be made abroad. In one survey a remarkable 77% of final-year university students in Zimbabwe said they faced family pressure to emigrate. Elsewhere there is evidence that medical faculty advise students to migrate in search of better training and to achieve their personal goals.[8,9]

Many people go abroad for training that may not be available in their own country, and many return home afterwards. Sri Lanka, as a matter of good practice, wants all its higher trainees to spend 2 years abroad learning their speciality. Other governments send trainees to specialist centres where they do not have local facilities. UK qualifications are in high demand in India and UK institutions still provide much of the educational infrastructure in former British Colonies. The Royal College of General Practice, for example, accredits all family doctor training in Southeast Asia, with the exception of Burma, in association with local bodies. The Royal College of Obstetricians and Gynaecologists has half its members from abroad.

A Chinese doctor gave me a personal slant on this when he told me "We learn our trades abroad and are now putting them to good use at home. When I returned home 5 years ago there were chicken coops, now there are multinationals."

These educational links provide some counterbalance to the damage done by migration and could, as I will argue, be built on much more strongly than at present to help increase the health workforce in many countries.

Figure 4.2 summarises some of the main push and pull factors for individuals.

Push	Pull
No jobs	Greater opportunities
Low pay	Higher pay, can send money home
Poor housing, schools etc.	Better opportunities for families
Poor work environment	Professional fulfilment
Family pressure	Active recruitment
Unsafe environment	

Figure 4.2 Push and pull factors

Some governments that want valuable hard currency sent home by their citizens working abroad actively encourage this migration. Of Ghana's GDP, 13% comes from such remittances, so I was not surprised that the former Minister of Health advocated such an approach to me when we met in 2006, suggesting that the UK might want to set up a planning agreement to do so.[10] Overall, remittances from migrant workers in all sectors to developing countries stood at US$72.3 billion in 2001 and were much higher than aid and development support.[11]

Cuba has a long history of exporting doctors, partly for humanitarian purposes and partly for economic reasons; in 2000, for example, they agreed a trade of 'doctors for oil' with Venezuela.[12] A further agreement in 2005 provided for the training of 50 000 medical personnel in Venezuela and the creation of 1000 free medical centres. Oil shipments to Cuba increased to 90 000 barrels a day. Many in Venezuela have welcomed this, although a BBC News Report of 15 July 2005 reported that Venezuelan doctors protested strongly that these incomers were taking their work away. The powerful trades unionism of the profession is as evident in poorer countries as in richer.

The story of the Philippines is often quoted. It is a remarkable example of a country that has taken the initiative. It has very deliberately chosen to export its labour and, as Patricia Santo Tomas, formerly Minister of Labour and currently Chair of the Philippines Development Bank explains, "manage the potential damage to our country from the migration of health workers". Four countries – Japan, the Netherlands, Norway and Denmark – have established training schools in the country and, at the time of writing, the Philippines has agreements on recruitment with 82 countries.[4] Other countries, such as Egypt, train far more doctors than they can afford to employ. Ethiopia is now planning to do the same.

At the moment, and in the round, it seems clear that the costs of migration outweigh the benefits. However, any cost–benefit analysis involves making judgements about the value of the benefits and some countries, as we have seen, have chosen to export their trained health workers in return for specific benefits in cash or kind.

Figure 4.3 summarises the main costs and benefits to a country from the migration of some of its health workers.

There are many factors 'pulling' people as well. Some rich countries actively encourage the import of health workers; others have, knowingly or unknowingly, allowed it to happen. In my own country, the UK, the establishment of the NHS in 1948 was accompanied in the following years by a big increase in demand for services and a big increase in costs. Looking at the circumstances of the time I don't think it was the costs of training that drove the government of the day to support such large-scale immigration of health workers, but rather the shortage of trained health workers for the NHS.

The UK Government wanted to deliver on its promise of a universal health service for all its people. This promise drew in health workers from what were then its colonies, with the Caribbean providing many nurses and South Asia many doctors. It is clear that the NHS could not have prospered without this immigration.[13]

Other countries may not always have made such explicit promises; although there is little doubt that if the new US administration does promise to widen access to healthcare to bring in currently unserved parts of its population, it will create further demand for trained workers. Even without such promises, rich countries need to keep meeting the

Costs and benefits of international nurse migration

Costs	Benefits
Brain and/or skills drain	Educational opportunities
Closure of health facilities due to nursing shortages in a given area	Professional practice opportunities
	Personal and occupational safety
Overwork of nurses practising in depleted areas	Better working conditions
Potentially abusive recruitment and employment practices	Improved quality of life
	Transcultural nursing workforce (e.g. racial and ethnic diversity)
Vulnerable status of migrants	Cultural sensitivity/competence in care
Loss of national economic investment in human resource development	Stimulation of nurse-friendly recruitment and contract conditions
	Personal development
	Global economic development
	Improved knowledge base and brain 'gain'
	Sustained maintenance and development of family members in the country of origin

Figure 4.3 Costs and benefits of migration for exporting countries. From Kingma M. Nurses on the move: historical perspective and current issues. *The Online Journal for Issues of Nursing* 2008; 13. Available at: www.nursingworld.org/MainMenuCategories/ANAMarketplace/ANAPeriodicals/OJIN/TableofContents/vol132008/No2May08/NursesontheMove.aspx

rising demands for health care, which come from their increasingly older and more prosperous electorate.

The new patterns emerging

The patterns of migration are, however, not standing still and there is now plenty of evidence that the global movement of trained health workers will increase as the newly rich countries of the Gulf, South Asia and increasingly India and China demand a greater share of this scarce resource. They will draw health workers from rich countries as well as poor, which in turn will put more pressure on the poor.

Singapore is an interesting case in point. It only recognizes the qualifications of doctors trained in five countries – the UK, USA, Canada, Australia and New Zealand – and actively recruits from them all. Singapore and other South Asian countries such as India and Thailand cater for the growing demand for high-quality healthcare from people who are willing to travel to obtain international standards and can afford to do so. Singapore is within 7 hours' flying time of 40% of the world's population, 2.5 billion people. It and its competitors can anticipate a growing market and will need the staff to deliver.

The Gulf States, too, are hungry for people. I am indebted to Dr Elsheik Badr from the Sudan for information about what is happening in the Gulf States and its likely longer term impact. He explains that in these six countries with a population of about 35 million, two-thirds of whom live in Saudi Arabia, around three-quarters of both doctors and nurses already come from abroad and the proportions as well as the actual numbers are set to grow further.

Dr Badr is understandably concerned about the impact on his own country. The Gulf States have a preference for Arab-speaking Muslims. Of Sudanese doctors who match these preferences, 10% are already there. The number of those training suggests that the flow will increase. Saudi Arabia is training less than 900 doctors a year for a population of around 20 million, whilst the Sudan trains four times as many for a population double the size. Dr Badr describes very clearly the factors that make the Gulf States attractive. There are many 'pull' factors – geographical proximity; language, social and cultural similarities; a suitable environment for families; policies promoting expatriate labour; good remuneration and active recruitment. Sudan, sadly, has in recent years provided more 'push' factors than 'pull' with internal conflict, lack of stability and a weak economy continuing to push people away.

This discussion has concentrated on doctors, in part because there is better information available on their numbers and their movements. There are overlapping patterns for other groups of health workers. Many nurses have migrated from their homelands. I was told by Government officials in India that they expect to lose about two-thirds of the nurses trained there within 2 years of graduation. There may, however, be a changing pattern here as well. Dr Badr has noticed that recently the Gulf States want more nurses than before as their health services develop and more care can be given. As more sophisticated services develop in other countries and as nursing itself raises its profile and status we can expect this new pattern to develop.

It is far harder to analyse migration patterns for other disciplines because of the lack of information and, frequently, the lack of common definitions of roles and professional boundaries. Singapore, which only recognises medical qualifications from five countries, sets no limits at all for the other groups of health workers outside nursing and medicine. They allow, for the moment at least, a multiplicity of different professions and standards to flourish unregulated in these areas.

These new patterns are aided enormously by improved communications and technology. The international recruitment agency mentioned earlier has seen a very large increase in enquiries about migration and in actual movement in the last 5 years. It believes that a significant part of this is due to the ubiquitous Internet and its 24-hour-a-day capability to roam the world. Like everything else, health worker migration has speeded up.

Ethical policies for international recruitment

These new pressures from the newly prosperous and rapidly growing parts of the world add to those being experienced in the already prosperous parts with their ageing populations. Migration has continued apace along the old routes and through the old connections as pressures to increase health staffing are continuing. Some estimates suggest that the USA will require 1 million more nurses in the next 10 years.[14]

In 2000 the UK, once again as in 1948, set out on an ambitious plan to improve the NHS and, once again, required a massive increase in staffing. As Chief Executive I oversaw a planned growth in staffing in the NHS by 250 000 from 1.1 to 1.35 million in a 5-year period to 2005.[15] Our strategy this time was threefold: to train more health workers ourselves, to bring people – mainly women who had left to have children – back into nursing and to recruit internationally for staff who would fill some of the gaps whilst we trained our own. Our aim over time was to be self-sufficient in staffing. We also brought into healthcare for the first time many more people as helpers, assistants and technicians to support the work of professionally trained staff.

Our strategy was very successful. The NHS was able to deliver on almost all its planned improvement targets, thanks in part to these new staff. By 2007 the increased number of UK graduates whom we had trained was coming into service and the UK became very largely self-sustaining in terms of education and training.

The UK had come under serious criticism from African countries, led by South Africa, in the late 1990s and had developed both an ethical international recruitment policy and, later, a code of practice. It subsequently signed an agreement with South Africa to support each other's health systems through the exchange of information and personnel for mutual benefit. As a result of this agreement, around 330 doctors and other health professionals from the UK went to work in South Africa for periods between 2002 and 2005.[16]

Almost 30 000 of the UK 250 000 increase in staffing came from international recruitment with the rest generated internally. The ethical policy and code of practice meant that we tried very hard to take health workers only from countries with a surplus and where their governments supported the recruitment. To this end we signed agreements with the Philippines, Spain and countries in eastern Europe and saw a large increase in staff from some of these countries. Most of the 30 000 indeed came from these countries, but not all.

Whilst the ethical policies had a significant impact, some people found ways around the rules. Some recruiters working for private sector health companies continued to recruit from other countries. Once in the UK, it was comparatively easy for health workers to switch to the NHS.

There were also many sad cases of foreign doctors, particularly from South Asia, who had heard via the media or family members that jobs were plentiful in the UK and spent all their savings to come to the UK in search of their fortunes. Many more than were needed came and the vast majority never found jobs. In the end we posted advertisements in a number of Indian cities to discourage health workers from coming to the UK in order to try to halt this flow.

When the increased output from training at home started to come through, the UK tightened its immigration rules and made nursing no longer a 'shortage speciality' in 2006, a designation which had brought with it relatively easy entry to the country in earlier years. This finally made immigration to the UK very difficult for health workers from outside the European Community. The flow of nurses from South Africa fell from its height 2114 in 2002 to 39 in 2007.[17]

However other doors were open in other countries for would-be migrants and, crucially, any global recruitment policy and code of practice must aim to address the 'push' factors as well as the 'pull'.

The UK ethical policy and code of practice was seen as a milestone by many and much of the African criticism of the 1990s turned into the desire to see this as a forerunner of more such policies and codes in the 2000s. At the same time ethical policies and codes were developing in different parts of the world, for example, in the South Pacific and Latin America; whilst the Commonwealth, with its large African membership created a code of practice in 2004.

The pressure from low- and middle-income countries, which were generally the source of all this migration continued to grow, and in 2004 the World Health Assembly passed resolution 57.9 that, amongst other things, called for the development of a global code of practice on the international recruitment of health personnel.

As a result the Health Worker Migration Global Policy Advisory Council, chaired by the former President of Ireland, the Honourable Mary Robinson, and Professor Francis Omaswa from Uganda, was established to review existing practice, collect ideas for implementation and propose a global policy and code. The Council, of which I am a member, has supported the World Health Organization in designing a Code of Practice that is expected to be put to the World Health Assembly in May 2010.

This code, for the first time, aims to bring together all aspects of international recruitment and seeks to address the roles and responsibilities of all parties – the source and destination countries, the recruitment agencies, the employers and the health workers themselves. It is, of course, focussed on the damaging drain of skills and talent from poor to rich countries, but it also seeks to address the wellbeing of migrants and tackle abuse and exploitation.

The code, if passed by the Assembly, will be voluntary and can't by itself deal with all the problems. It will, however, set out the clear expectations of the world health community and have the moral authority and standing to help all those who in their own countries are struggling to manage the effects of migration and improve the lives of migrants. It will be a major step forward in making improvements.

The Code does not directly address the issue of whether poor countries could and should be compensated by the rich for training health workers who subsequently migrated. There have been many demands for this. The simple notion that a country should compensate another for every health worker that moved from one to the other fails to come to terms with the practical difficulties as well as the political difficulties of implementing such a scheme.

At the practical level, all sorts of questions arise from how to trace a worker though the complex patterns of migration to the question of who should compensate whom for the postgraduate training received abroad by a migrant who brings their new skills home to serve their native country. The political issues are also complex, with some recipient countries simply not willing to discuss compensation and others wondering why they should compensate countries that fail to provide health workers with good working conditions or, worse still, persecute their citizens.

There are other approaches. In the USA, in 2005 Senator for Illinois Richard J. Durbin introduced a draft Bill in the US Senate to compensate Africa for the contribution of African workers in the USA through a series of grants and projects. The Bill never progressed in the Senate but does show that other ways of looking at the question of compensation are possible.[18]

In the UK, in 2007 I recommended in *Global Health Partnerships*, a report to the then UK Prime Minister, Tony Blair, that the UK should recognise that it has responsibilities as a global employer because so many of its doctors and nurses were first trained abroad. I argued that, as part of that responsibility, it should support a massive scaling-up of training, education and employment of health workers in developing countries. The UK Government did not quite accept this in its formal response to my report. However, it did say that it would be supporting international efforts to scale up the education and training of health workers in developing countries and has, indeed, done so.[19]

Norway appears to be going further down the same route. It commissioned a report in 2005 on its likely health workforce needs by 2030 and, whilst it did not identify a precise level of increase in the report, concluded that it needed many more people working in health and social care just to keep up with an ageing population, let alone to raise standards.[20] Private conversations suggested the total increase needed might be 30% or more. They set out their ambition to achieve this growth in a way that did not affect poor countries.

Following further deliberation and debate Norway has declared a moratorium on international recruitment and is considering proposals to increase its support for the education and training of health workers in poor countries in recognition of the fact that we now have a global market place for trained health workers and a global interdependence in health.

Norway seems set to move beyond the Code and take positive steps to intervene in the world market for skills and experience. This must surely be the important next step. The Code can help dampen migration and manage its ill effects, but wider interventions are also needed.

The health crisis

There is a wealth of evidence and anecdote that shows that today's approaches are failing and we have a real crisis on our hands that affects rich and poor countries alike. There is a critical shortage of health workers worldwide. It is not a local problem for poor countries but a global crisis that affects us all.

It is not just a health worker crisis. It is a health crisis. There are about 1 billion people in the world without healthcare. Around another billion have minimal access to help and support. This means that, in the absence of sometimes quite simple help and advice, thousands die or are disabled from preventable and treatable causes. These thousands of individual tragedies are a tragedy for us all.

It is worth asking whether trained health workers make a great deal of difference. Intuitively one would expect that having health workers able to give advice and even simple treatments would help improve health and save lives. The evidence shows they do. Trained health workers with the right skills in the right place at the right time reduce levels of maternal mortality and increase child and infant survival as Figure 4.4 shows.

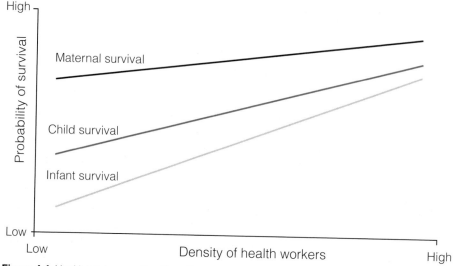

Figure 4.4 Health workers matter. From World Health Report 2006 - working together for health. Figure 1 – health workers save lives, page xvi. Available at www.who.int.whr/2006/en/

There are many other factors, of course, that contribute to improving health such as the education of women, improvements in the environment and the availability of drugs and equipment. Our health is determined by much more than health systems and health workers, as earlier chapters have shown. More health workers will not be sufficient by themselves to improve the health of a population, but they will certainly be a significant and necessary part of any wholesale improvement.

The World Health Report in 2006 estimated that the global shortage amounted to at least 2.35 million doctors, nurses and midwives (or 4.3 million health workers of all sorts), with poorer countries worst affected. It calculated that 57 countries were in crisis: 36 in Africa, seven in the eastern Mediterranean, six in South East Asia, five in the Americas and three in the western Pacific.

The Report's figures cover the whole range of health workers from clinicians to pharmacists to laboratory workers and to those responsible for feeding patients and handling the logistics of supplies and equipment maintenance. All are in particularly short supply in the poorest countries.

The World Health Report based its estimate on assessing the increase in numbers that would be needed to enable 80% of women to have a skilled attendant at birth. This is a standard that is well below what would be seen as acceptable in high-income countries but far higher than existed in most low-income countries. A higher standard would require even higher numbers of workers.

We are a long way from achieving even this standard and it is clear that the wonderful ambitions of the Millennium Development Goals will not be achieved without large increases in trained health workers. Policymakers, nationally and internationally, are increasingly turning their attention to tackling this problem.

The staffing crisis

Whilst migration is a major factor, it is only one of many problems in ensuring that there are sufficient health workers to deliver improved health and improved services in poor countries.

If every one of the 135 000 African doctors and nurses were to return home, Africa's health problems would not be solved. The World Health Report estimates that Sub-Saharan Africa requires 1.5 million more health workers than it has currently to reach the minimum standard where skilled workers are available for 80% of deliveries.

The biggest single factor is that not enough health workers of all kinds are being trained. This applies in almost every country in the world as the following few examples show.

Until 2007 Ethiopia trained between 150 and 200 doctors a year (or about 2 per million of its population).[6] If all these doctors had stayed in the country they would now have to look after a population of about 80 million. A recent review of 12 Sub-Saharan African countries showed that at present rates of training it would take 36 years to reach the WHO's target of 2.28 health professionals per 1000 population and that some countries would never reach it.[21]

There is also a considerable variation amongst richer countries. The UK is now one of the few countries that train enough doctors for their own employment, with almost 8000 students a year (or about 125 per million) and 160 000 actively working doctors.[22] By contrast, the USA trains about 18 000 a year for a population of 320 million (or about 56 per million: half as much as the UK) and has about 900 000 doctors currently active.[23] Low levels of training are a problem both in richer and in poorer countries.

The pattern with nurses is also hugely variable. India trains about 10,000 per year for a population of 1.1 billion, compared to the UK's training of 25 000 for 60 million.[24] Zambia trains 1200 and estimates it needs to train 2100 to meet the needs of its population of 12 million.[25]

Training is not enough by itself. Health systems and health employers also need employment and operational policies that counter the 'push' factors described earlier. Poor working conditions, poor pay and employment conditions, the lack of drugs and equipment all need to be confronted. They not only push many health workers to emigrate, they persuade others to leave the health sector altogether.

This push to other sectors also applies, if less dramatically, in rich countries. When we in the UK wanted to encourage more women to return to nursing after having children, we found that the biggest factors were often that the working conditions didn't match their needs. We had to become very flexible and offer daytime and even termtime-only contracts, part-time jobs and crèche facilities.

Poor working conditions, employment and pay all contribute to health workers leaving government employment in the general services of a country and moving internally to work for the NGOs, the not-for-profit and the for-profit healthcare providers and suppliers. This movement, often bitterly resented by health ministries, contributes to the fragmentation of services and a concentration on the priorities that NGOs and outside donors see as important. The general health of the population may suffer as a result.

Underpinning many of these problems is the lack of money. Funding restricts the numbers of health workers that can be employed, their pay and conditions and the quality of their working environment. Shifting and short-term funding promotes the sort of 'churn' we see as health workers move from one organisation to another or from one country to another in pursuit of jobs and higher wages.

A further financial constraint in several poor countries has been the role previously played by the International Monetary Fund. It has taken the view in many countries that public spending, even for the development of human capital through health improvement and education, must be curtailed as countries struggle for economic stability and search for the holy grail of growth. This short-sighted and narrow policy has been very damaging in some countries and, even though the policy is changing to an extent, has left a legacy of destruction and bitterness. In some countries such as South Africa and Kenya there are unemployed health workers unable to find jobs in health care as a result of these policies.[26]

These human resources issues – of too few people being trained, concerns about pay and employment conditions as well as the working environment and the lack of money for health – affect people in some way in almost all countries of the world. In richer countries there are added complications arising from inbuilt rigidities in the way health workers are trained, employed and regulated.

There has been a continuing trend towards ever greater specialisation in the USA in particular but also in many other rich countries. This specialisation combined with greater regulation has led to peaks and troughs in the demand and supply of highly trained health workers. We have seen, for example, specialists in the countries becoming redundant as the demand for their skills shifts. A particular example in recent years has been in cardiac surgery, where many more patients who might previously have required surgery are being treated medically by cardiologists.

Specialisation and regulation also tend to increase costs and, in a world with shortages in crucial groups of health workers, there is rapid wage inflation. Dr Badr reports how the Sudan has doubled the pay of doctors but that, given the huge differences in what they can earn abroad it has made little if any difference in the retention of doctors. Other countries in Africa, too, are thinking of or have doubled doctors' pay, thereby using up significant sums from the nation's health budget.

This is a global labour market and it is helpful to look for the insights of economists in order to understand some of the dynamics. This chapter has shown how demographic, political and economic factors have driven up the demand for trained health workers in rich and rapidly growing countries. It has painted a picture of massive flows in many different directions as 'pull' and 'push' factors tug or thrust people into movement.

These sorts of discussions are often couched in the language of what is needed in a country with little reference to what can be afforded. Richard Scheffler a professor of health economics and public policy from the Goldman School of Public Policy at the University of California has recently brought just such an economist's insight to bear and generated a new model of the supply and demand for doctors globally, where he uses demand to mean what can be and is afforded in a country. This may be very different from models like the one WHO suggest is needed there.

Scheffler's model generates some different patterns with oversupply in some countries – where they can't afford to employ their own medical graduates – and undersupply in others where actual economic demand is unmet. Interestingly, it shows an oversupply in some richer countries. He uses this analysis to challenge conventional thinking.

Scheffler argues, for example, that the USA is not suffering from a shortage of doctors – rather, we are seeing the results of decades of misguided public policies. These policies have created a healthcare marketplace that often fails to deliver the right number of doctors, of the right specialty, in the right locations. Healthcare reform, Scheffler argues, is not just a matter of training more doctors. What the USA needs is a reform of healthcare policy that will spur the development of an efficient, cost-effective, and high-quality healthcare system.[27]

These arguments take us on to the questions of what sort of health workers do we need and want. Do poorer countries need to have the same sort of staffing structures as richer ones? Do richer ones need the traditional model, and can they afford it?

Conclusions – a global vision

This chapter has shown that the supply of trained health workers is truly a global health issue and needs global attention and some global regulation if the poorest countries in the world are not to suffer. Individual countries will not solve it by themselves. Three things stand out clearly amidst all this complexity. Firstly, there is now a very largely free and unregulated labour market in trained health workers that is creating instability in rich countries as well as poor. Secondly, it is the poor countries that suffer from the migration of health workers. Thirdly, the current situation is unsustainable.

The key question is very simple: how can poor Africa staff itself and how can rich Norway staff itself if we stick to the traditional approaches we know and understand? To answer this we need to create a new vision of what the world could be like if we didn't have this global instability and the accompanying and highly damaging export of valuable people, with all their skills and talent, from poor countries to rich. This vision would be based on three foundations:

- Our understanding that in terms of our health we are interdependent – our national success or failure in combating disease and improving health affects us all internationally.
- The free movement of ideas and people – and the opportunities to train and work abroad – will help us all in our shared quest for better health.
- We need a shared commitment that each and every country must have a safe minimum level of health workers to meet the needs of its population.

The Health Worker Migration Global Policy Advisory Council set out just such a vision in its submission to the WHO on the code of practice.[28] This vision – of interdependence, free movement and universal minimum standards sets out the direction we must travel. We also need to know how to get there.

We have already seen some of the steps we must take. We need international codes of behaviour to provide a shared framework of rules and expectations, whether they be about international recruitment or, as we will discuss in the next chapter, intellectual property. We need massive increases in the education and training of health workers – with rich countries supporting the poor. We need improvements in both employment and working conditions.

Underneath it all there is a global problem of resources. It is inconceivable that every country will be able to staff itself in the same way as is done in richer countries and even here, as we have seen, there is demand for ever more staffing. We need therefore to go further and redesign the whole way we conceive of health and deliver healthcare. We need to change the design of our healthcare systems and of our health workforce. We also need to understand what technology can do for us when trained human time will be at ever more of a premium. In conversation, Ruth Levine, of the Centre for Global Development, has taken this insight further and suggested to me that we really need to measure productivity in health services in terms of labour used not money expended. Human time is the real measure of expenditure in a service that is dependent on human skills and human caring.

Many countries and many planners have adopted an approach generally called 'task shifting' – the transfer of tasks from a more expensive staff group to another less expensive one – as a means of making scarce skills and resources go further. This has often been done with some reluctance and the expressed opinion that this is a second class way of doing things that will be abandoned when more money is available.

I will argue, however, that this very profession-centric view of the world misses the point. We need to train people to do the tasks that need doing in any country and not just to meet the needs of the professions. Nurses may well do some things currently done by doctors better than they do them, as well as more cheaply. Technology can help improve both quality and cost. Perhaps most importantly, the patient and community also have potentially the most important roles of all.

This redesign brings profound changes for the professions and for their education and training. It will be an important part of moving on from the existing conception of western scientific medicine and helping make it fit for the twenty-first century. However, before we explore these changes, we need to look at the other side of the unsustainable import–export business, the import of ideas to poor countries from the rich.

The next chapter describes the modern Race for Africa. It concentrates on the actions of the rich world and the impacts of its ideas and activities in poor countries. It also begins to show, however, that poor countries are beginning to create their own ideas and to create their own new designs to deal with the health problems that they so well understand.

References

1. International Labour Office. *Report of the Committee of Migrant Workers, Provisional Record 22.* 92nd Session, International Labour Conference, Geneva, Switzerland, 2004.
2. Clemens MA, Pettersson G. New data on African health professionals abroad. *Human Resources for Health* [Online]. 2008, **6**: 1. Available at: www.human-resources-health.com/content/6/1/1.
3. Marchal B, Kegels G. Health workforce imbalances in times of globalization: brain drain or professional mobility? *Int J Health Plann Manag* 2003; **18**(Suppl 1): 89–101.
4. Health Worker Migration Global Policy Advisory Council Meeting: conference proceedings, September 18–19, 2008, Marlborough House, Commonwealth Secretariat, Pall Mall, London, UK.
5. Kaba AJ. Africa's Migration Brain Drain: The costs and benefits to the continent. [Online]. USA-Africa Institute. 2004. Available at: www.popline.org/docs/1671/298662.html.
6. *Ethiopian Medical Journal* January 2008. Volume 46, Supplement 1.
7. Dumond JC. Health Workforce and Migration: An OECD perspective. Sixth Coordination Meeting on International Migration. United Nations, Population Division, 26–27 November 2007.

8. World Health Organization. *The World Health Report 2006: Working together for Health.* 2006.

9. Hagopian A, Ofosu A, Fatusi A et al. The flight of physicians from West Africa: Views of African physicians and implications for policy. *Soc Sci Med* 2005; **61**: 1750–60.

10. Addison EKY. *The Macroeconomic Impact of Remittances in Ghana.* Bank of Ghana, 2004. Available at: www.g24.org/Addison.pdf.

11. The World Bank. Global Development Finance: Striving for stability in development finance. 2008. Available at: www.worldbank.org/prospects/gdf2003/tocvol1.htm.

12. Calvo-Ospina H. Cuba exports health. 2006. *Le Monde Diplomatique.* Available at: mondediplo.com/2006/08/11cuba. [Accessed 5 August 2009].

13. Department of Health. *Many rivers to cross – the history of Caribbean contributions to the NHS.* Available at: www.manyriverstocross.co.uk/index.html.

14. US Department of Health and Social Services. Health Workforce Studies. Available at: bhpr.hrsa.gov/healthworkforce/.

15. The NHS Information Centre. *Staff in the NHS 2005: An overview of staff numbers within the NHS in England 2005.* Available at: www.ic.nhs.uk/webfiles/publications/nhsstaff/NHSStaffNHSLeaflet240406_PDF.pdf.

16. Paper HMM (E) (OG) INF3 for the Commonwealth Health Ministers Meeting, May 2006.

17. The Nursing and Midwifery Council: Statistical Analysis of the Register.

18. Krauss K. Senator Durbin and others introduce bold measure to tackle massive health worker shortage in Africa, fight AIDS. *Physicians for Human Rights.* 2007. Available at: physiciansforhumanrights.org/library/news-2007-03-07.html. [Accessed 25 September 2009].

19. Crisp N. *Global Health Partnerships: The UK contribution to health in developing countries.* 2007. Available at: www.dh.gov.uk/en/Publicationsandstatistics/Publications/PublicationsPolicyAndGuidance/DH_065374.

20. Directorate of Health and Social Affairs. Recruitment of health workers: towards global solidarity. 2007. Report to the Ministry of Health and Care Services, Norway. Available at: www.helsedirektoratet.no/vp/multimedia/archive/00018/IS-1490E_18611a.pdf.

21. Kinfu Y, Dal Poz MR, Mercer H, Evans DB. The health worker shortage in Africa: are enough physicians being trained? *Bull World Health Organ* 2009; **87**: 2225–30.

22. From Medical and Dental Schools Register. Inspected 22 Oct. 2009.

23. US Deparment of Health and Human Services, Health Resources and Services Administration. *Physicians Workforce Policy Guidelines for the United States, 2000–2020.* 2005. Available at: www.cogme.gov/16.pdf.

24. Khadria B. *International Nurse Recruitment in India.* Health Services Review 2007 June: 42 (3pt2) 1429–1436.

25. Ministry of Health, Government of the Republic of Zambia. *Zambia National Health Strategic Plan 2006–2010.* Available at: www.who.int/nha/country/zmb/Zambia_NH_Strategic_plan,2006-2010%20.pdf.

26. Kingma M. Nurses on the move: a global overview. *Health Serv Res* 2007; **42**: 1281–98.

27. Scheffler RM. *Is There a Doctor in the House?: Market signals and tomorrow's supply of doctors.* Stanford, CA: Stanford University Press, 2008.

28. Health Worker Migration Global Policy Advisory Council Meeting: Conference Proceedings Sept. 18–19 2008, Marlborough House, Commonwealth Secretariat, London, UK.

5 Unfair trade (2) – importing ideas and ideology

I was the wrong person with the wrong question at the wrong time.

As the Mozambique Minister of Health entered the small committee room with his officials in tow I could see immediately that he was cross, very cross. We were at the World Health Assembly in Geneva in 2006 and I had requested an interview in order to ask him what more the UK should be doing to help improve health in Africa.

I don't know where he had just come from. I now wonder if he had been sitting all morning in meetings where he and his African colleagues had felt patronised by people from rich donor countries telling them what they should be doing; perhaps he was merely suffering from too many hours of long speeches and the interminable time wasting of that great Assembly.

Upright, smartly dressed and very articulate, he let me know from the outset that he was fed up with being told what to do by foreigners. He understood his own country very well, thank you. He knew what his priorities were. Did I understand that the international agencies providing pills for immunisation were only doing part of the job? What use was a pill if a child didn't have any clean water to swallow it with? He didn't care if immunisation was their priority. He wanted help with infrastructure, water, roads, schooling and employment. He didn't want to be told what he should be doing.

This, my first meeting with Minister Paulo Ivo Garrido, reminded me of the story I had heard about one of his predecessors as Health Minister for Mozambique, who had naturally assumed that on taking office he would be responsible for the health of his population. He discovered, however, that he was really the Minister for health projects which, he paused for effect, were run by foreigners.

It also underscored very clearly what it felt like to be a recipient of foreign aid. Mozambique, in common with other countries, received aid from many individual countries, including the UK, from international agencies and from many NGOs, small and large. All of them gave aid on their own terms and all of them wanted it monitored against their own criteria. It is only a small step from here to telling people what to do.

This problem is not unique to Africa. Many countries receive more than 100 separate monitoring visits a year, two or more per week, and have to write reports for all their donors. Some countries need to devote half the precious manpower of their ministries of health to dealing with foreigners and 'projects run by foreigners'.

It must have been very galling for the Minister. I learned, as I got to know and respect him at later meetings, about the passion and energy he brought to the role. Unlike many, he was in the post for the long term and, as a surgeon, understood healthcare well.

For my part I got far more from the interview with the Minister than I had expected, being, as I was, forcefully reminded that aid and development are also about power and about who sets the agenda and, of course, about who is accountable to whom.

This story sets the scene for a chapter in which I describe some of the ways in which ideas and ideologies are imported from richer to poorer countries alongside aid, trade and other relationships. It is very important to stress at the outset that very many of these ideas are extremely beneficial: scientific knowledge, technical knowhow, commercial and governmental understanding are all immensely valuable. However, like all good things, they bring their own problems, some of which get in the way of progress. This chapter concentrates on this darker side.

Power is at the heart of this, with the ability it gives richer countries and institutions to impose their ideas, intentionally or unintentionally. It has as its social and psychological accompaniment what I call here an 'unconscious superiority', which affects the way people think and behave.

The chapter looks first at how power influences economic relationships – aid, trade and investment – and also shapes the way healthcare can be delivered by influencing what problems can be addressed and how this will be done. It goes on to look at some of the psychological aspects that have led, amongst other things, to undervaluing local knowledge and neglecting context and circumstance.

The chapter concludes by arguing that accountability needs to be reversed if aid and international development are going to have lasting impact. People need to ask Minister Garrido for permission to work in his country and for his approval for what they are doing, not the other way round.

The new race for Africa

There is a new *Scramble for Africa* underway.

We start by looking at how aid, trade and investment are being used in the global competition for influence and access to natural resources.

In the eighteenth and nineteenth centuries the European great powers competed for territory and resources around the world. They wanted the best harbours and the best marketplaces from which to control the trade routes and secure the diamonds and the gold and other metals waiting to be unearthed in the vast interior of the continent.

They divided Africa up between them, leaving a legacy of language, religion and law and a continent of nation states constructed around the boundaries of their conquests and treaties rather than on Africa's own heritage of peoples and kingdoms.

The contest sprang to life again in the twentieth century, but this time it was much more about influence, with the communist and non-communist worlds buying the favours of the 'non-aligned' newly independent states of Africa with investment and aid, arms and hospitals. Marxist–Leninist philosophy flourished in a variety of local forms, far distant in every sense from its northern birthplace, whilst right-wing dictators, hardly distinguishable from their communist neighbours, lived well under western protection.

Today, the new great powers of China and India use different weapons to compete with the Europeans, Americans and Russians for natural resources as well as influence. Both these countries, themselves recipients of development aid, provide aid and investment in their turn to other countries. China in particular has been generous with its help for major infrastructure projects, often in return for access to mineral deposits, seaports and open markets for its vast manufacturing output.

In this century, the total amount of investment into Africa has overtaken international aid for the first time, with China playing a major role.[1] It is no wonder, therefore, that there was such a good response from African countries when they were invited to Beijing in November 2006 to discuss friendship and development. Out of a total of 53 African heads of state in the continent, 41 attended. As many or more are expected at this year's gathering.

All this aid and investment has not yet made the recipient countries rich and is unlikely to do so at the present rate of progress. The common thread throughout all this competition is power and the way that international relationships are almost always skewed in favour of the rich and powerful. International treaties, international organisations, infrastructure projects, trade deals and the way aid is given all reflect power relationships. They all help to maintain the status quo.

Aid itself provides a good example. It is often linked with trade so that a good part of the money given in aid returns to the donor in payment for goods and services. This happens in three main ways: the first, which we have already touched on, is that the aid given is tied, directly or indirectly, to a trade deal or to access to resources of some sort.

The UK alone amongst the largest countries has since 1997 had a rigid separation between trade and aid, with its Department for International Development (DFID) required by law to spend development money only on the relief of poverty and without reference to the UK's trade interests. Others have no such scruples and aid is seen as a legitimate part of both foreign and economic policy. Money may be given, for example, for a dam or a hospital on condition that a company based in the donor country builds it or that permission is given for mining.

The second link between aid and trade is that aid money itself may be returned directly to the donor country to buy services. In 2006, research by the charity Action Aid showed that one-quarter of the aid provided by rich countries, or US$20 billion a year, funds expensive external technical assistance such as consultants, research and training instead of going directly to the countries concerned. Expatriate consultants typically cost around US$200 000 per year; more than one-third of this is spent on school fees and child allowances.[2]

The third link, which has now been to some extent broken, was the provision of loans, which over time left poor countries owing vast sums to richer ones. Many developing countries are engaged in debt relief programmes and to date 24 countries have obtained debt relief through the Highly Indebted Poor Countries Initiative (HIPC) and Multilateral Debt Relief Initiative (MDRI).[3] Nevertheless these schemes are controversial among some developing countries and international NGOs because to qualify for debt relief schemes countries must adopt adjustment and reform programmes suggested by the IMF and World Bank.

The result of all this is, as Figure 5.1 suggests, to reduce the amount of aid countries actually receive.

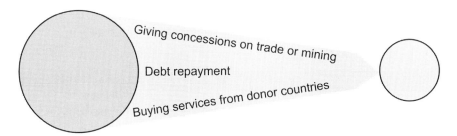

Figure 5.1 Shrinking aid – the costs of receiving aid reduces its value

Today, when trade, aid and investment have replaced colonialism and shared ideology as the main basis for the relationship between the rich and poor countries, the actual terms of trade are little, if anything, more favourable than they ever were.

Richer countries are better able to lobby and influence others in international negotiations and have the financial resources to sit out disagreements. The Doha Free Trade negotiation, which might have done something to reduce the disadvantages poor countries face in their trade with the rich, has been quietly abandoned. The European Common Agricultural Policy, which protects small farmers in rich countries, remains largely unreformed. Richer counties can find many different ways of being protectionist.

Many poorer countries have relatively little bargaining power because they produce very few goods for export; some only have one crop or product. They are very vulnerable to global price swings in copper, tobacco or coffee, or whatever their particular product is, as well as to mood swings amongst rich consumers over tastes and concerns about 'food miles'.

Despite the international commitment to make trade work for Africa there has been little change and it has only 3% of the world manufacturing exports and 2% of the world's commercial services.[3] The World Trade Organisation has established a Task Force on *Aid for Trade* in order to promote further trade growth, although the results are not yet apparent.[4] It is a very similar picture with regard to inward foreign investment. Richer countries get the bigger share. In 2007, two-thirds of global foreign direct investment went to developed countries.[5] The top three recipients were the USA, the UK and France.[5]

The short-term outlook makes the picture even gloomier. The World Trade Organisation has predicted that global trade volumes will decline by 9% during 2009 as a consequence of the global recession[6] with low-income countries worst affected as richer countries contract their commitments and become more protectionist. It has been estimated that Africa, for example, has lost US$50 billion in growth alone.[7]

The economic crisis presents the world with a choice between on the one hand stimulating investment and consumption within the rich countries and, on the other, promoting a new 'new deal' that addresses the investment needs of the whole world, promoting stability and real world growth. It is a choice between pessimistic protectionism and hopeful ambition.

Figure 5.2 shows the relative size of aid, foreign direct investment (which is about 20 times greater) and trade (which is more than 100 times greater). It demonstrates how important aid is to the poorest countries in the world. It also suggests, however, that the greatest prize for them and other developing countries will be to increase their share of

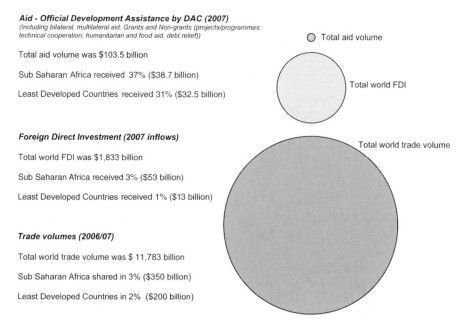

Aid - Official Development Assistance by DAC (2007)
(Including bilateral, multilateral aid. Grants and Non-grants (projects/programmes, technical cooperation, humanitarian and food aid, debt relief))

Total aid volume was $103.5 billion

Sub Saharan Africa received 37% ($38.7 billion)

Least Developed Countries received 31% ($32.5 billion)

Foreign Direct Investment (2007 inflows)

Total world FDI was $1,833 billion

Sub Saharan Africa received 3% ($53 billion)

Least Developed Countries received 1% ($13 billion)

Trade volumes (2006/07)

Total world trade volume was $ 11,783 billion

Sub Saharan Africa shared in 3% ($350 billion)

Least Developed Countries in 2% ($200 billion)

Figure 5.2 Aid, trade and investment – some key figures for 2007. From UNCTAD WIR 2008; UNCTAD LDC Report 2008; OECD 2007; WTO 2007

foreign investment and of trade and thereby grow their economies. They need bigger slices of the two bigger cakes.

Importing ideas and ideology

The international financial and economic institutions have faithfully reflected these power relationships and adopted the ideas and ideologies of the powerful countries that created and continue to control them. For the best part of three decades from the 1970s the Bretton Wood Institutions, led by the International Monetary Fund (IMF), required countries that sought their help to introduce 'structural adjustment' policies.[8]

These policies, based on a liberal free market view of the world were designed to ensure that developing countries had sound financial systems that would encourage private sector investment and the development of commercial activity. One consequence of this was very often a requirement to cut government expenditure. This in turn led to reduced spending on health, education and social development, which was seen as non-productive and, in the short term at least, not a priority for economic development.[9]

There is continuing controversy as to the precise impact of these policies. The main point here is that they undervalued the importance of investing in health and education and the consequences of not doing so. One direct result was damage to the retention and recruitment of health workers as salaries were frozen or decreased and investment in tertiary institutions was reduced.

The negative consequences of these policies remain today with unemployed nurses in Kenya laid off or unable to be recruited in the public sector as a result of a government hiring freeze in response to the IMF, and nursing schools closed in other countries for the same reason, whilst countries desperately need trained health workers.[10]

In southern Africa, in particular, the resulting damage to health and social development was enormous at a time when AIDS was already beginning to kill a generation of productive workers and throw millions into destitution. The authoritative Commission for Africa recognized these problems and recommended renewed investment in higher education and universities in order to re-build the infrastructure that was needed.

The IMF has the responsibility, with the World Bank, to help stabilise economies in difficulties and to work with countries to achieve sustainable growth. This means it must continually balance social expenditure with growth and affordability. Too often is was seen to get the balance wrong and, most tellingly, to ignore the contribution that health and education make economically through building what economists call 'human capital'. This is the very human capital made up of healthy productive workers that, coupled with financial capital, is needed to drive the engine of the economy.

Some of today's criticism of the IMF may be unfair and based on its old practices or on the wishful thinking of those who believe investment in health and education is itself such a long-term good that short-term economic consequences are unimportant. The Centre for Global Development, an independent think-tank, undertook its own review of the IMF in 2007 and concluded that it could and should do much more to promote social development without compromising its credibility.[11]

Now 2 years later, more radical reforms appear to be needed if developing countries are to achieve the Millennium Development Goals. The old economic and financial institutions created after World War II have not served us well in our financial crisis. The time has come to turn the world upside down, get rid of the old orthodoxy and think afresh about what we are trying to achieve.

There is a sense, as I write, that we are using the weapons of the last war to fight the next one.

Power also sets the health agenda

In health, as Minister Garrido understands too well, power sets the agenda. Ideas and ideology come with the money. It is no surprise that donor countries impose explicit conditions on how money is spent. In 2005, for example, the UK required Malawi to make basic health services free to all its citizens as a condition of a massive investment in staffing and health infrastructure.

It shouldn't come as a surprise either to know that donor countries don't all want the same things. The USA, by contrast, promotes health insurance and, by implication, wants users to pay some of the cost of their own healthcare. Each country it seems, exports its own beliefs about how health services should be run, regardless apparently of the success or failure of those policies in their home countries.

This is not in itself a new trend. Former British Colonies from Hong Kong to Jamaica have health services modelled on the British NHS and for a long period their medical and nursing schools had many expatriates on their staffs. This legacy lives on in the thousands of young professionals who have come to the UK for their training and who still aspire to membership of one of the UK Royal Colleges.

Medical staff from former French Colonies can tell a similar story and exhibit the same high level of pride in their graduation from a French University and their years of training in Paris or Lyon or Marseilles. They, just like the South Americans or Filipinos trained in the US system, take home with them a share in the experience and worldview of their teachers and mentors.

More problematically, we have seen the intrusion of current domestic politics into international development. Two linked issues, birth control and abortion, have heavily influenced American policy, provoked a split with many other donors and slowed progress on improving death rates amongst women and children as well as on AIDS.

Domestic American politics meant for years that US aid officials were unable to embrace the full ABC of AIDS prevention, where A stands for abstinence, B for be faithful and C for use a condom if the other two do not apply. They have in many cases been forbidden to promote condom use or other forms of contraception outside marriage because to do so has been considered to be condoning or even encouraging immoral behaviour.

I now hear many of my American friends saying that, with their new Administration, they will once again be able to re-join the world community, sign up to the treaties and come to the table.

It is even more important, however, that it is a different table with more seats and better amplification for the voices from the poorer and less powerful countries.

Vertical power

Another major development in recent years has been the way in which international organisations and donors have come together to tackle the major health problems. UNAIDS, which brings together 10 UN agencies to confront HIV/AIDS was set up in 1994 under the leadership of Peter Piot. We have subsequently seen the introduction of the global health initiatives: the big international funds set up in partnership by a consortium of donors to tackle one or a small number of diseases such as the Global Fund for AIDS, Tuberculosis and Malaria (The Global Fund) or Global Action on Vaccination and Immunisation (GAVI). The USA, presumably wishing to maintain its own identity as a donor and thereby emphasising its separation from the rest of the world, has also set up its own version in The President's Emergency Plan for AIDS Relief (PEPFAR).

These bodies have very large sums of money at their disposal. The Global Fund's budget for 2008 was US$177 million; GAVI's was US$697.7 million; whilst PEPFAR had US$5.4 billion to spend during the same year. These bodies, also known as 'vertical funds' because they take a single aim and pursue it down through the system making sure that everything is aligned to achieve the aim, have generally been very successful in their immediate aim. GAVI, for example, has directly or indirectly ensured that 213 million children have been immunised for the period 2000–2007.[12]

Sir Richard Feachem and Professor Michel Kazatchkine, the successive Directors of the Global Fund, rightly claim great credit for ensuring that more than 2 million people in

Africa are now receiving Anti-Retroviral Therapy (ART), the treatment that keeps AIDS victims alive.[13] Their organisation has, however, been criticised for the very vertical nature of the Global Fund and the way in which in pursuit of its aims it ignores and sometimes damages other services. Like PEPFAR, it is accused of ignoring the potential for working with other services, poaching their staff by paying higher wages and dominating and distorting the whole health system in a country through the sheer amount of money that it is able to bring to bear.[14]

Their dominance is shown by the single example of Zambia, where in 2006 the PEPFAR spending of US$150 million was higher than the total government budget for all other health services of $136 million.[15]

Vertical funds, whether these enormous global initiatives or the smaller versions often run by NGOs, undoubtedly have had some negative effects. If any issue or disease is given priority status it will mean that others are given lower or no priority and treated accordingly. It is the nature of priority setting. I know from my own experience of running the NHS in England that it can be very difficult to keep a balance between the priority services and the rest and that it is not possible to have priorities and pretend that you can treat every service equally. The real criticism is that more could be done both to ameliorate the bad effects and to contribute to strengthening the local health system.

I went to see Mark Dybul, then the Head of PEPFAR, to discuss this early in 2008. We had met before and I had previously been struck by the calm and thoughtful manner in which he discharged his very large and complex role. He is a US Admiral and, because he was shortly to attend a state occasion with the President, met me dressed in his formal blue uniform complete with silver buttons and braid. We sat beside the large American flag in his office whilst, courteous and informal as ever, he talked me through the issues.

Mark was one of those people who work at the point where power meets practicality. He had to reconcile on a daily basis the demands of the politicians and the needs of patients. He was directly accountable to the President and dependent on Congress for every dollar he spent. His budget had been voted as an Emergency Fund for AIDS and Congress expected every dollar to be spent on AIDS and on nothing else. As a doctor, experienced and knowledgeable about working with AIDS patients in poor countries, he had a deep understanding of the problem on the ground and of what needed to be done.

He told me about what he was already doing to counteract any problems that PEPFAR might be causing and help strengthen health systems more generally. He had opened his supply chains to other organisations, so they could deliver other drugs and equipment. He paid for the training of health workers who did more than just work on HIV/AIDS. He funded shared facilities and clinics. He pointed out that his local staff did work with others, took account of local conditions and had a measure of flexibility within the overall framework set by President and Congress.

We discussed what could be done about the fact that PEPFAR could pay health workers more than they would get from local organisations and that as a result existing health services lost people to PEPFAR and, perhaps even, had to close. It was obviously an important freedom for his organisation and meant that it could be confident about employing people to deliver the services his Congress required. Nevertheless he was open to ideas to limit the freedom and to make some recompense by training more people locally.

As a result of our discussion The Global Health Workforce Alliance recommended that any foreign organisation working in a country should commit to keeping staff pay and conditions broadly in line with local rates and contribute to paying to train more health workers locally. Whilst this recommendation still needs to be implemented, it is important both because it ameliorates the problems that can be caused by vertical funds and because it introduces a notion of accountability to the country where the work is taking place.

Figure 5.3 gives a very simplified version of the dilemma that vertical funds have faced in trying to deliver their goals, whilst supporting the local health system. On the positive side their focus can lead to quick results; but on the negative side, it can inadvertently lead to damaging other services.

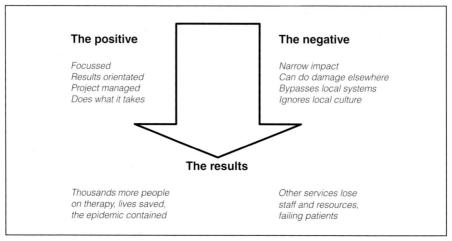

Figure 5.3 The paradox of vertical power – how to maximize the positive impact whilst minimizing the negative effects

Whilst the threat posed by the big communicable diseases dominated thinking at the turn of the century, attention has now switched to the need to strengthen health systems. Long-term success in tackling communicable diseases as well as non-communicable diseases and securing the safety of mothers and children depends on having a working health system in every country in the world.

The massive global vertical funds are adapting. GAVI now explicitly funds health system strengthening whilst the Global Fund spends around 25% of its budget on human resources. In the longer term it has been suggested that the Global Fund and PEPFAR might widen their remits and, even, become general global funds for health.[16,17]

In 2009 there has been a concerted attempt to bring together these global vertical funds with the health systems-strengthening initiatives. It looks as if Ambassador Eric Goosby, Mark Dybul's successor at PEPFAR, will be have the freedom to pursue a much wider agenda than Mark was able to do.[18]

This vertical approach is, however, also used by many much smaller NGOs. Less well resourced, they may nevertheless also do damage at the same time as they are doing good. They too need to tackle this paradox of vertical power and minimise the negative effects whilst maximising the positive impact.

Multiple requirements from multiple sources

The vertical funds represent one source of the import of ideas to poor countries. Top down and focussed, they encapsulate a particular notion of how improvement can be delivered. In doing so they make assumptions about how citizens and professionals alike behave and about how health systems need to be organised.

Over the same time period we have seen a spate of health reforms being introduced around the world that adopt a very different, and rather more horizontal, model of change. Often inspired by the World Bank or one of the big consulting firms, they take an economist's perspective and seek to influence behaviour. They concentrate on incentives for citizens and for providers, aim to generate more funds mainly through insurance and advocate mixed public and private systems of clinicians, clinics and hospitals.

Sometimes the vertical fund and the more horizontal incentives-based system are brought together as, for example, in Rwanda, where the Global Fund works closely with a developing insurance system in an effort to build a functioning health system whilst at the same time tackle the scourges of AIDS, TB and malaria.[19]

Other factors and other players complicate the mix. New philanthropists, most notably The Bill and Melinda Gates Foundation, have come on the scene to join the many existing bodies with proud records such as the Rockefeller Fund and China Medical Board. The Gates Foundation through its sheer scale – it spent about US$1.7 billion in 2007 – is able to influence other donors as well as implement huge programmes of its own.[20]

The problems of multiple donors with multiple priorities and multiple monitoring requirements have been recognised internationally for years. The Millennium Development Goals, which 189 countries signed up to in 2000, was both a statement of intent and a powerful means for unifying priorities.[21] From this point onwards there has at least been agreement on the top priorities.

The Paris Declaration of 2005, signed by more than 100 countries, moved this forward by setting out principles for working together. These principles cover the importance of country's owning their own development plans, alignment of international efforts, harmonisation of processes, results orientation and mutual accountability.[22]

More recently there have been a number of new groupings set up to put these principles into action and help coordinate action in different ways. These have included a regular H8 meeting that brings together eight of the most powerful international health organisations,[23] the Campaign for the Health Millennium Development Goals launched by the Norwegian Prime Minister and other global leaders to help keep a focus on the Goals,[24] and the International Health Partnerships (IHP) launched by the UK Prime Minister to create a single agreement between a country and its multiple donors.[25]

As I write, the UN meeting on the Millennium Development Goals in New York in late September 2009 has brought together world leaders around these issues. There are signs of a better coordinated approach with the global initiatives playing their part, the new US Administration fully participating and the promise of longer term and more stable funding. It is a promising moment; progress appears to have been made.

In the meantime, some idea of the complexity of relationships that countries must currently manage is revealed in Figure 5.4, which shows the Ministry of Health (MOH) in one country almost buried by its helpers. Money comes with strings and here they form a hopeless tangle that can trap the country in bureaucracy.

All of the initiatives to improve the situation have made some progress. However, wording is open to interpretation, aid and investment overlap, governments change and, perhaps most importantly, many countries and organisations are not signed up to these processes. The USA, Japan and France, to take only three examples from amongst the long-term donors, are not part of H8, the Campaign for the Millennium Development Goals or the International Health Partnerships.

Moreover there appears to be reluctance by these long-term donors to collaborate with China, India, Brazil or the Middle Eastern countries that are now entering the arena and vice versa. There appears to be a tendency to keep each other at a distance rather than a willingness to share their knowhow or experience. China in particular is having a major impact in Africa and rehabilitating and building hospitals and health centres such as Luanda General Hospital in Angola.[26] There is surely an opportunity for collaboration here.

These arrangements, which look deeply confusing and confused to any casual observer, must be a source of great frustration to anyone, like Minister Garrido, who is trying to make things happen in their own country. This picture, to exaggerate only partly, is one of many many governments and organisations doing what they want to do and cooperating when it suits them.

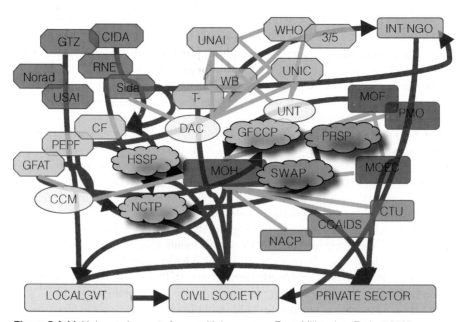

Figure 5.4 Multiple requirements from multiple sources. From Millennium Project 2005

There appears to be no notion of accountability to the recipient country and its people with all the governments and organisations looking homewards to their populations, Parliaments and Boards for direction and accountability. The power relationships are all one way. It is clear who makes the decisions. Recipient governments can challenge the donors; some, the most powerful, do and a very few low- and middle-income countries, like Cuba, choose to stand outside this whole framework of relationships. Most, however, need the money and accept the deal on offer.

Donor governments are, of course, accountable to their parliaments and people and will want to take credit for their work; however they could nevertheless find ways to be more accountable to the recipients. The UK leads the field in providing 'budget support' whereby they do give aid directly to a government to support its plans. Whilst this goes a long way towards recognising that countries 'own' their own plans, the reality is that the money still comes with strings and involves an enormous amount of negotiation and authorisation.

Another route, already touched on, which would compliment budget support, would be for donors, of all sorts, NGOs as well as governments, to seek approval for their plans from the government to work in their country and pay a levy of, say, 15% of expenditure as a contribution to training or wider health infrastructure. It would be a sort of licence to operate in the country.

This arrangement, which would turn the current one upside down, would have its own difficulties. It couldn't be applied everywhere and, if badly handled, would build an awful bureaucracy and could create appalling opportunities for bribery and moral blackmail. However, the principle of accountability it embodies is the right one and a simple scheme could be devised whereby organisations pay a simple levy to an infrastructure fund in, say, the 20 poorest countries.

If we take the example of both the Global Fund and PEPFAR paying 15% of their Zambian expenditure to support the training and employment of people in the general health services of the country, they would boost expenditure in these areas by far more than 15% and undo any collateral damage the vertical funds might do in the ordinary course of their work. The new proposals from the September 2009 UN meeting would mean that they would be supporting systems-strengthening schemes; this approach, however, would mean that they had to leave the decision making to the country.

Perhaps it might also be possible to devise a way in which recipient countries were able to assess the performance of the donors. Would it not be possible to create a system for measuring the waste that occurs through the duplication and fragmentation of donor efforts and for assessing the effectiveness of donors on this basis?

Unconscious superiority

Power, as we have seen, influences global economic structures and relationships and the way healthcare is supported globally. There are also social and psychological aspects to be considered. The power relationship is embedded in behaviour and attitudes amongst donors and recipients alike.

It is easy to see continuity here with colonial times. The structure of health services and thinking about healthcare has been very much influenced by its origins. Healthcare was organised primarily for the colonialists and the local elite, with the majority of people looking to local healers and missionaries for help.

After independence the new rulers continued broadly with the same institutions and structures and built central and regional hospitals, and very often continued to look towards the former colonial power for leadership. Outlying areas were still left to traditional healers and missionaries. Traditional medicine itself was ridiculed or ignored, observed but not studied, and certainly not really taken seriously until the last decade. The colonialists had left, but their ideas remained.[27]

Professor Barbara Parfitt has written extensively about how western nurses unconsciously apply their own values and prejudices in their work in developing countries. I met her, perhaps appropriately for the topic, in the UK's House of Lords. In a richly decorated room with paintings of famous British sea victories on the wall, the atmosphere redolent of history, power and empire, we discussed how the attitudes and values of British nurses, formed over many years, were exported around the world.

Barbara had herself worked for long periods in developing countries and, as she explains in *Working Across Cultures,* noticed how some nurses were able to achieve a great deal and others, apparently as well skilled and motivated, very little.[28] She noted the traps nurses could fall into in their unconscious assumptions about their patients and the power of western medicine and, most particularly, that they could set up an unhealthy dependency relationship with their patients and the whole local community.

The problem, put simply, was that the nurses with their western ways and skills became too powerful. They ignored and thereby disempowered traditional knowledge and skills and became the sole possessor of knowledge and the only one who could help.

This problem is, of course, familiar to clinicians and patients in rich countries, where it is easy for a confident and capable nurse to become the expert on my health and, as it were, to own my problems and my solutions. This is, as we have seen in Chapter 3, a very powerful theme in western medicine whereby the professionals own the whole process and practice of healthcare with patients being not just patient, but totally passive. Commercial organisations reinforce this dependency with the often mysterious, to the layman, power of their potions and treatments. The problem is far worse, however, where there is an in-built power relationship as there is between the trained western clinician and the uneducated local person and where a culture of deference to graduates and professionals may enhance the effect.

Barbara has subsequently developed a model to show how nurses can understand and manage their own behaviour and help create a more collaborative and sustainable approach to health.[29] It reminded me of the way another clinician had approached a similar problem in the very different circumstances of New York.

Dr Mauvareen Beverley works in Queens in a hospital that draws its patients from the wide range of people of different ethnic backgrounds in the poorer parts of the Borough. She and her colleagues had learned from years of experience that handing out prescriptions and giving advice to their many patients with chronic illnesses didn't work for many people. Many of their patients simply didn't take their medication or follow their treatment regime.

The hospital staff knew that they needed to work alongside their patients if they were going to succeed. They also knew that a part of the problem was with themselves as clinicians. They had all learned to be culturally sensitive in their time in healthcare and knew about the different cultures and faiths amongst their patients, but they still felt unable to connect fully with the patients they needed to reach. Their power and knowledge was, they knew, part of the barrier.

In a story that combines humility with determination, Mauvareen told me how they devised a new short programme for their front-line staff that helped them both to understand their patients more deeply and to find ways to ask the right questions and make the right interventions. It was no good just being culturally sensitive; as Mauvareen put it, you needed to act as well.

The values, beliefs and knowledge of the clinician are potential barriers to care and independence in multicultural London, Paris, Toronto and New York just as they are in poor countries. They reflect the dominance of western scientific medicine and the power it lends its practitioners.

Copying the rich

So far in this Chapter I have described the way ideas and ideologies are passed on from the dominant rich countries to the poor. It is a top-down process that reflects where power sits. However, it is equally apparent that people in poor countries want many of these imports. People want western medicine. They can see it works. People want to be doctors and to enjoy the income and status it brings. Their extended families want to share in their success. Equally, many countries have taken on those secondary characteristics of medicine as a profession, which, as I argued in Chapter 3, can be so useful but can also be so damaging to health.

They have embraced a far-reaching idea of professionalism and the need for regulation to the extent that doctors and their trade unions are even more powerful than they are in rich countries and that strict regulation, for example in South Africa or Brazil, means that only doctors can carry out tasks that are done by other health workers in the UK, France or the USA. This is a closed shop.

Many have also wanted to show that they, too, can have facilities, services and expertise every bit as good as the West. There was a particular tendency at the time of independence for African countries to invest in hospitals and prestige services within their capitals when, in reality, the biggest need was for primary care and public health spread throughout their country.

A variant of this, which has had longlasting detrimental effects, was the way that Ethiopia changed its medical curriculum in the 1980s to an American model. Previously its curriculum was based much more on primary care and public health and geared to the needs of the country. Now it turns out graduates who understand the specialities and the needs of western environments and who are, therefore of course, ideally suited to emigrate to Washington, take their Board exams and add to the 'brain drain'. It is only in the last few years, that with inspired local leadership they have reversed this process and started to create a local curriculum again.

This desire to compete with the West is still evident in some places today. I visited one country in Africa where the Chief Executive, himself a doctor, and his senior doctors took me round the main hospital in the second largest city. It was a large site with ward blocks and departments spread throughout the grounds. Each block had two wards, one on top of the other, each of which consisted of a large open area with around 30 beds, a small treatment area and open lavatories. At a rough count, I could see that there were about 60 patients in each ward, some on the floor and some on the beds, and about an equal number of relatives and friends. More were camped outside.

It was a dismal and depressing scene of the kind too often found in Africa. The blocks were discoloured concrete, the grounds full of rubbish. At one end there was a large tip of discarded equipment, much of it looking as if it had been donated from richer countries. There was surprisingly little noise given the number of people who sat and stood around, following our little group with their eyes. It wasn't a particularly hot or humid day, but the buildings stank.

The Chief Executive showed me where a new Emergency department was being con-structed with US$50 million provided by the Government. He said it would have a heli-copter landing pad and be equipped to international standards. He also told me proudly of the new cancer centre they had just opened and of his plans to increase the range of specialities.

In the cancer centre, new and not yet in use by patients, the lead doctor gave us a hor-rifying slide show made up of pictures of his patients. All of them had enormous tumours on different parts of their bodies; one with a tumour growing from his shoulders almost the size of a second head. It was sad, depressing and, I thought, unnecessary. Only later did I understand why he had done it.

My wife had been following at the back of the group and talking to the doctors there, just out of earshot of the Chief Executive. The cancer director told her that he had a hope-less task. There was so much to do in cancer in his country, but he couldn't do it in the cancer centre. He wanted to be working more closely with local services in the town and the countryside, tackling prevention, diet and, where possible, early diagnosis. Here, in his new centre, he would only get the hopeless cases, the people he could nothing for, the people with the enormous tumours, the people in the slide show.

The obstetrician told her a similar story. He desperately wanted the funding to train and support workers in the countryside, who could help look after mothers, identify problems early and get them to his hospital. Instead he felt stranded where he was, receiving too many patients who were too late to save, already too far gone in bleeding to death when they ar-rived in his care. The precious money was all going into the hospital and not the services.

Later we saw the cancer doctor in a bar in town. He asked me to try to change the Government's plans and help set up a locally based service that would address the real needs of the population. Back in the capital my comments were clearly unwelcome. It was too late; the money was committed.

This simple story helps illustrate the complicated nature of the problem. Here was a country taking a western model and applying it inappropriately to its own circumstances. It was both ironic and tragic.

The irony was that western planners faced with anything like this position would al-most certainly have tried to develop a community-based solution. The tragedy was, as we saw in Chapter 2, that almost 30 years earlier an international consensus was established at Alma Ata that the most effective way to improve health in poor countries was to invest in community-based services and primary care. It simply didn't need to be like this.

Learning to listen

This chapter presents a fairly depressing picture. The rich and powerful world still exerts a huge influence on its former colonies. It still controls the levers of power in the world. It still gets the better part of the deal in trade negotiations and still finds ways to exploit the natural resources, human and physical, of the poor countries in the world.

Turning to health, we export our ideas and ideologies to poor countries alongside our aid. We introduce our beliefs about western medicine, about how you organise health services and about how you get things done. We accompany them with our values about life and society and freedom. We reinforce them with our behaviour and our attitudes. We exercise an unconscious superiority. We explain and educate. We make demands about structures and organisation. We tell people what needs to be done. We set the agenda.

The effect of all this is to overpower other ideas and beliefs and to encourage people to copy the things that have made us so successful in the past and to adopt our winning strategies. These things are so powerful precisely because they have been so successful. Western medicine with all its accompanying science, professionalism, commerce and vast expenditure has, as I have argued earlier, been astonishingly successful. However, as I have also argued, it is now beginning to fail us because it is unable to handle the complications of context and society and the complexities of human behaviour.

The power is so overwhelming that it can stop us thinking about context and society. We can, if we are not careful, discount the differences between societies: ignoring how women and children are treated, ignoring the corruption and forgetting that the very poor live lives of such fragility that any setback becomes a catastrophe. We can simply fail to realise that an idea that works so well at home may be completely irrelevant elsewhere.

The force of our ideas is, in effect, so noisy that it can stop us listening to other perspectives.

This can quite literally be the case. Over the last 3 years I have been in many meetings discussing health in poor countries and planning action for improvement. In many cases there has been a majority present from the rich world and, although I have not done the analysis, I am quite sure that the minutes would reveal that many more words were spoken from that perspective.

This can be very uncomfortable for all concerned as the lonely African or Asian finds themselves by turn expected to speak for all developing countries or simply ignored. It is very easy, if you are looking for it, to catch the exchange of glances between people from developing countries as others are speaking and, just occasionally, to see them group together to press a point.

I remember one meeting with 15 of us present, two of whom were from Asia and two from Africa, when my Pakistani neighbour, a very distinguished clinical academic, turned to me and said "Go on Nigel, back the developing countries on this one." He was making explicit a hidden split that is there in many meetings.

It is very easy to see how this happens. Organisers have an extraordinarily difficult job in setting up international meetings and making sure that they get good people to attend. They can always find another well-educated and articulate North American or European and, because there are so many of them and they are richer, they are more likely to be available and able to travel. It makes it even easier, of course, if the meeting can be held in North America or Europe.

Listening is two way, of course. There needs to be dialogue between all parties, with the points of view and knowledge of people from richer or poorer countries listened to and evaluated on its merits.

Is it all a waste of time?

It is little wonder that some people have looked at all this and concluded that aid doesn't work, that international development is a waste of time and that western interference in the affairs of poor countries is just that, interference.

There is a considerable charge sheet to answer. This chapter has exposed three of the main charges: that what really matters is economic growth not aid, that aid is wasteful and bureaucratic; and that aid builds dependency. We will examine each in turn but will start with the most damning claims of all: that governments haven't kept their promises and that aid doesn't work anyway.

Global Health Watch, which has set itself up as an unofficial watchdog, offers a very wide-ranging assessment of the ways in which the international community has failed to deliver on its promises to provide more money and describes how, where money has been provided, it has failed to use it to make the necessary impact. The ONE's DATA Report similarly demonstrates that many governments simply haven't done what they promised and rates countries on their performance: with some doing slightly more than they promised and most striving to meet targets or falling far behind.[30]

These analyses serve the very useful purpose of publicising performance and thereby holding governments to account to public opinion. Global Health Watch also draws out the importance of the underlying power and economic relationship between donors and recipients and argues that the existing model for international development, which doesn't address this imbalance, is flawed. Aid won't help if at the same time trade deals systematically undermine a country's ability to grow its economy and raise its people out of poverty.

It is worth at this point returning to the discussion in Chapter 2, where I argued that to improve health it was necessary to do three things at the same time: (1) tackle the health problems directly; (2) alleviate poverty and its associated problems: and (3) change the way that national and international social, economic and political structures, between and within countries, get in the way of improvements. They keep the rich rich and the poor poor. They maintain the status quo.

Using this framework and the discussion in this and earlier chapters it is possible to put together as in Figure 5.5 a rough score card for the impact of aid and international

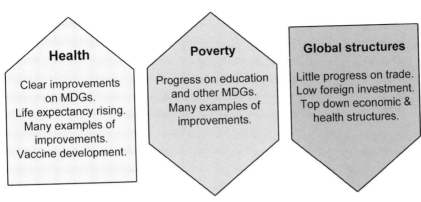

Figure 5.5 Aid and development – a rough scorecard

development on health. I believe there has been progress on the purely health aspects, some improvement on poverty but little on changing global structures.

There are problems in holding governments to their promises and failures in delivery, but there has been undeniable progress in tackling the specific health issues and in dealing with some of the problems associated with poverty. However, as I said at the outset, the criticisms in this chapter should not make us lose sight of the remarkable progress that has been gained by using the knowledge, the science and the economic strength of richer countries. Moreover, it has been very impressive to see the way that many world leaders have continued to press this agenda, even at a time of financial crisis. As a citizen of the UK, it is good to see that the UK Government has so often been at the forefront.

People may disagree with the particular assessments I have made in the table, but no one, surely, will disagree with the fact that it is the social, economic and political structures and imbalances that are now the biggest obstacles to progress.

Global Health Watch, like others, describes essentially the same problem as I do and suggests that we need a new model for development that rebalances the relationships between the richer and poorer countries of the world. The argument in this chapter supports their analysis but, as we shall see, takes it further by arguing that we need to go beyond the ideas of development and think instead about how we are all now so much more interdependent and need to develop together or not at all. The idea of co-development needs to replace the concept of international development.

It's the economy, stupid!

Looking at the particular charges on the charge sheet in turn, they all have some validity. The first is the very simple assertion that all you need for development is economic growth. People who take this view point out that the astonishing rise of several countries in Southeast Asia was not due to aid and development support. China, they add, has taken more people out of poverty through economic growth in the last 10 years than all the development activity in the rest of the world put together.

Dambisa Moyo, herself an African and an economist, has argued that aid and development create dependency and give support to poor national leadership and government and that other countries should stop interfering altogether in the affairs of poorer countries. They should be allowed to stand on their own feet and develop themselves in their own way within a global free market.[31]

These arguments are very important in emphasising the role that economic growth can play in development, promoting the idea that countries have to take responsibility for themselves and countering any notion that external aid and international development support is sufficient. However, in their simplest form they misinterpret both history and the current environment.

Any analysis of the successful growth of these economies shows that there were many factors responsible for the growth including government activity, protectionism and foreign investment. Many too, including China, have been the beneficiaries of aid. Other commentators critique the argument that free trade and open markets are enough by pointing to the fact that today's rich nations built their economic empires on very different and much more protectionist approaches. Rich countries that advocate a simple free market approach are in effect 'pulling up the ladder'.[32]

The picture that is presented is too simple. It also ignores the present reality that growing protectionism and reducing global trade are making the position harder for poorer countries to grow and that, even if growth comes eventually, their populations have health needs today. Their health needs, as we have seen elsewhere, are important to us all.

Nevertheless economic development must surely take centre stage and the illustration on p 86 of this chapter that shows the relative sizes of aid, foreign direct investment and global trade clearly demonstrates how important it is for developing countries to get access to the investment and the trade flows they need to grow.

The invention of international development

The earlier description of the multiplicity of donors is pretty damning and lends credence to the assertions of some critics that aid is wasteful and bureaucratic and serves only to create an industry that benefits thousands of people from the richer countries. This chapter has hinted at something of the extraordinary amount of activity that goes on internationally around development and aid.

There are meetings, conferences, assemblies, planning sessions, reviews, monitoring visits and liaison between donors and recipients, between donors and donors and between regional and national groupings. It is the domain of economists and policymakers who mix politics with their professional analysis as they dispense vast sums of public money.

There is waste, there is bureaucracy and both must be tackled; but there is also a wider problem embedded in the very notion of international development. This is the implication it so often carries of people doing things for other people, of knowing better, and of there being somehow a clear distinction between developed and developing countries.

We have invented this massive infrastructure, or perhaps more accurately superstructure, of international development and used it to capture everything to do with the development of a country. It now deals with everything from the global economic issues of trade and financial stability to the detail of education, agriculture, health and transport.

They are, of course, all connected and it is very important that someone has the overview and the whole picture. Moreover I have constantly been impressed by the quality of the people working in this field. However, in bringing together all these topics there is a danger of losing focus on the important detail of each one and of the things we share.

Taking health as just one example, it is clear that development agencies and the associated think-tanks and universities have become the experts on international development and health. Agencies and government departments employ many such individual experts. However, they are not necessarily the experts on all aspects of health; who, as one would expect, generally work in health services and in other parts of universities.

Governmental and organisational structures reinforce this separation. Departments for international development find it very hard, in my observation of a number of western countries, to draw on the expertise in their own country. They have their own internal experts and it is only occasionally, as with the threat of pandemic flu, when the country itself feels threatened that the whole government structure – from Health Department to International Development, Foreign Affairs Ministry and Treasury – pulls together around a global health problem. More often than not it is the development experts who talk about health systems and health worker training from a theoretical point of view, without having been involved recently with these issues in their own country.

Our structures continue to treat the health issues of other countries as if they were quite distinct from health issues in our own. It is the old world where academics talked of international health and meant the health of other people, rather than the new world, often characterised as being about global health, where we are beginning to understand just how connected and interdependent we all are.

In practice this separation can be problematic and Dr Paul Farmer rails against development experts in Africa, whom he has seen using sensitivity to local culture as a reason for not giving a child a medicine.[33] A sick child is still a sick child. He or she needs to be treated by a health expert, not an international development one.

He illustrates the wider point. Health issues are still health issues even if they are in poor and far away countries. We risk a great deal if we separate these poor countries off from the global mainstream. We will both be the poorer for it.

We must unfreeze our minds and think more clearly about international development and what it has become. The very success of inventing a new professional discipline may now be part of the problem. Putting it at its simplest and perhaps rather unfairly, do we need a model where development experts do all aspects of development or one where a far wider group of people, – teachers, farmers, engineers and nurses – use an understanding of development in their work?

Aid creates dependency

The psychological discussion earlier shows that there is a real risk of developing dependency; however, crucially, if we understand this better we can do something to mitigate its effects. This is by no means a hopeless task, particularly if we learn to listen better.

We could start by listening to individuals. There are many outstanding people in poor countries and many outstanding leaders. We could invite more of them to our meetings. We could listen better. We could find better ways to listen to the voices of the poor and try to understand why so many poor people 'define poverty as the inability to exercise control over their lives.'[34]

We could also try to listen out for and understand better the implications of the far-reaching changes underway in many countries. I have concentrated in this chapter on Africa and the poorest countries in the world and presented a relatively simple picture of the relationship between two groups, the rich and the poor. The reality is much more complex and far messier.

Power and influence are shifting and what, even 10 years ago, looked to the West like a fairly simple picture of high-, low- and middle-income countries with a one-way flow of aid and development, is now much more differentiated and complex. There are different power groupings, different flows of aid, different influences and different identities being forged.

Our relationship with poorer countries is not just about them and their needs. It is also about us and our needs. We are at a point when many people in rich countries are beginning to recognise the problems we have in sustaining and growing our health systems. We are reaching the limit with our current model. It needs major attention. This is our crisis too.

Recognising our own weakness in this way should make us more open to new ideas. It should also help us to support the development of poor countries better. It could, even, break down some of the barriers between developed and developing countries and help us as equal partners to learn and develop together.

Just as the idea of international health – the health of others – has been replaced by a shared notion of global health, co-development or global development, the development of equals, needs to replace the idea of international development.

The sting in the tail

We must also free our minds from some of the ingrained assumptions associated with western scientific medicine. These are very powerful, deep seated and difficult to challenge. This is nowhere better illustrated than by the current debate about 'task shifting'. This expression is used to describe the way in which some tasks previously done by one group of professionals such as doctors are shifted to another group such as nurses. Similarly, some tasks done by nurses might be shifted to other less well-trained groups.

It is often argued that poor countries can't afford to have many doctors and nurses and therefore every effort should be made to find ways to shift as many tasks as safely as possible to cheaper groups. Many people seem to see this as a purely temporary solution to be used only until the countries can afford the desirable level of staff. Nevertheless, a great deal of effort is now going into devising training courses and protocols to put this in place.

I remember discussing this in a meeting in Kampala when one by one the Africans in the room ridiculed the notion. Their complaint was not about unskilled people taking on these tasks, but about seeing the world purely in terms of the established professions. Why were we starting with the professions and deciding what would be done? Shouldn't it be the other way up? Shouldn't we decide what needs to be done and then decide who is best placed to do it? Or as they put it rather more forcefully, who do they think has been doing these tasks all along? Let them send us some doctors and nurses and we will gladly shift some tasks to them.

In unfreezing our minds, we need to look at what is happening elsewhere and think about how it applies to the rich world as well. BRAC, the massive Bangladesh NGO, is doing just that and is applying its learning in its home country to projects it is establishing in Africa, but also in the USA.

This chapter has been about what we import into poor countries from the rich. What if it were the other way round? What might we learn?

Ultimately it is the coming together of ideas from rich and poor countries that will have the most effect. In the next chapter we look at the lessons from poor countries, which, for the reasons we have discussed, largely go unnoticed or misunderstood, and with their wider significance unrecognised.

Conclusions

This chapter has described the many different ways in which ideas and ideologies are imported into poorer countries and illustrated how power dictates international relationships and shapes the way people think and behave. It has shown how these wider forces play out in health with the very top-down vertical funds, NGOs and donor countries all attaching their own strings to the aid they give with the result that there is much confusion and some harm, as well as improvement.

The chapter has suggested that some progress can be made in tackling these problems by improving accountability. It recommends that current processes of accountability should be turned the other way up so that any organisation working within a country must make itself accountable to the country and agree to contribute to the wider development of the health system and health infrastructure.

It raises the question of how to make sure that we don't put up artificial divides between health in richer and poorer countries. There is much to learn from each other, many of the issues overlap and we are increasingly interdependent. Should we not be talking about our shared health issues, and taking this further, not about development but about co-development?

References

1. Perry A. *10 ideas changing the world right now. Time Magazine.* Available at: www.time.com/time/specials/packages/article/0,28804,1884779_1884782_1884769,00.html.
2. Action Aid International. *Real Aid: Making Technical Assistance Work.* 2005. Available at: www.actionaid.org.uk/index.asp?page_id=100631.
3. World Bank. *Debt relief at a glance.* Available at: web.worldbank.org/WBSITE/EXTERNAL/NEWS/0,,contentMDK:20040942~menuPK:34480~pagePK:34370~theSitePK:4607,00.html.
4. www.odi.org.uk/iedg/aid4trade.html.
5. UNCTAD, United Nations, Geneva. *World Investment Report 2008: Transnational Corporations and the Infrastructure Challenge.* Available at: www.unctad.org/en/docs/wir2008_en.pdf.

6. WTO. *World trade 2008, prospects for 2009*. Press Release PRESS/554; 23 March 2009. Available at: www.wto.org/english/news_e/pres09_e/pr554_e.htm.
7. World Bank. *Africa likely to be worst hit by financial crisis*. April 23, 2009. Available at: web.worldbank. org/WBSITE/EXTERNAL/COUNTRIES/AFRICAEXT/0,,contentMDK:22154832~menuPK: 258649~pagePK:2865106~piPK:2865128~theSitePK:258644,00.html.
8. Riddell JB. Things fall apart again: Structural adjustment programmes in Sub-Saharan Africa. *Journal of Modern African Studies* 1992; **30**: 53–68.
9. World Health Organization. *Structural Adjustment Programmes*. Available at: www.who.int/trade/glossary/story084/en/index.html. [Accessed 29 September 2009].
10. Schuman M. Economist challenges recruiting hyperbole. *Can Med Assoc J* 2008; **178**: 253.
11. Center for Global Development. *Does the IMF constrain health spending in poor countries?* June 2007.
12. GAVI Alliance. *GAVI Alliance Factsheet*. 2009. Available at: www.gavialliance.org/resources/3EN_GAVI_ Alliance09_web.pdf.
13. The Global Fund. *Scaling Up for Impact: Results Report*. 2009. Available at: www.theglobalfund.org/ documents/publications/progressreports/ProgressReport2008_high_en.pdf.
14. *Global Health Watch 2: an alternative world health report*. Available at: www.ghwatch.org/ghw2/ghw2pdf/ ghw2.pdf. London: Zed Books Ltd; 2008.
15. Prakongsai P, Patcharanarumol W, Tangcharoensathien V. *Can earmarking mobilize and sustain resources to the health sector?* Bulletin of the World Health Organization 2008; **86**(11): pp. 817–908.
16. Jack A. Symptom to systems: How aid skews health services. *Financial Times*. [Online]. 27 September 2007. Available at: www.ft.com/cms/s/0/67c56088-6d26-11dc-ab19-0000779fd2ac.html. [Accessed 29 September 2009].
17. Ooms G, Van Damme W, Baker BK, Zeitz P, Schrecker T. The 'diagonal' approach to Global Fund financing: a cure for the broader malaise of health systems? *Globalization and Health* 2008, **4**:6doi:10.1186/1744-8603-4-6.
18. High Level Taskforce Report. *Maximizing Synergies between Health Systems and Global Health Initiatives: Initial Summary Conclusions*. Venice, July 2009; *Maximizing Synergies between Health Systems and Global Health Initiatives: Initial Recommendations*. May 2009.
19. The Global Fund. Available at: www.theglobalfund.org.
20. Gates Foundation. *Gates keepers: civil society voices on the Bill and Melinda Gates Foundation. Three points for Gates Foundation from non-American sources*. Available at: gateskeepers.civiblog.org/blog/ _archives/2008/11/21/3986465.html. [Accessed 29 September 2009].
21. United Nations. Millennium Development Goals. Available at: www.un.org/millenniumgoals/bkgd.shtml.
22. OECD. *The Paris Declaration and Accra Agenda for Action*. Available at: http://www.oecd.org/document/ 18/0,2340,en_2649_3236398_35401554_1_1_1_1,00.html.
23. First informal H8 Agency Meeting, July 2007, New York. More information available at: http://www. internationalhealthpartnership.net/ihp_plus_about_agencies.html.
24. World Health Organization. *Global campaign for the health millennium development goals: progress report*. [Online]. Available at: www.who.int/pmnch/topics/mdgs/noradprogressreport/en/index.html. [Accessed 29 September 2009].
25. DFID. *The International Health Partnerships launched today*. [Online]. Available at: www.dfid.gov.uk/ news/files/ihp/default.asp. [Accessed 25 September 2009].
26. Centre for Chinese Studies, Stellenbosh University. *China's Interest and Activity in Africa's Construction and Infrastructure Sectors*. November 2006.
27. World Health Organization. *Global health histories: Legacies of colonialism in African Medicine*. Available at. www.who.int/global_health_histories/seminars/nairobi02.pdf.
28. Parfitt BA. *Working Across Cultures: A study of expatriate nurses working in developing countries in primary health care*. Farnam, UK: Ashgate Publishing; 1998.
29. Parfitt BA. *The State of Global Health – Nursing and Midwifery: Offsetting negative influences of globalisation*. Oxford: Blackwell Publishing, 2006.
30. ONE International. *ONE's DATA Report 2009*. Available at: www.one.org/international/datareport2009/.
31. Moyo D. *Dead Aid*. New York: Farrar, Strauss and Giroux. 2009.
32. Chang, HJ. *Kicking Away the Ladder: Development strategy in historical perspective*. Bel Air, CA: Anthem Press, 2002.
33. Farmer P. *Pathologies of Power: Health, human rights, and the new war on the poor*, Berkeley, CA: University of California Press, 2003, p. 419.
34. Narayan D. *Poverty is Powerlessness and Voicelessness*. Finance and Development, International Monetary Fund. 2000. Available at: www.imf.org/external/pubs/ft/fandd/2000/12/narayan.htm.

6 Learning from low- and middle-income countries

Fazle Hassan Abed wanted to give me a simple message.

We were talking on the nineteenth floor of a building in Dhaka from where we could look out over the city. Just below us there was a U-shaped bend in the river, its base near the foot of the building with its arms extending away into the distance on either side. There were three- and four-story buildings along the outer sides of the U and one could imagine how in another city, or here at some future date, this would be a very attractive place to live with river walks and restaurants, their lights reflecting in the river at night.

At the centre of the U was a slum. It wasn't the largest or the worst slum in Bangladesh, but it was a slum nonetheless. We could see the temporary shacks made of wood and cardboard and plastic and between them the pathways that were no more than muddy channels filled with rubbish. There were more than 2000 urban slums like it in Bangladesh. They were the reasons BRAC existed.

I had come to meet the founder of BRAC in his headquarters and had just asked him how, based on his experience, the world could make faster progress in reducing deaths in childbirth and meet the Millennium Development Goal of cutting such deaths by three-quarters. He replied quietly and without the slightest hesitation: empower the women.

There was a long running argument in Britain in the late nineteenth century about when might be the right time to give working people the vote. On one side the reformers argued that they needed to be educated first, so that they would use it wisely. On the other, the radicals simply replied that if they had the vote they would educate themselves.

Mr Abed is with the radicals.

He told me later about how BRAC decided to launch a campaign in 1979 to teach families how to care for children with diarrhoea. They were aware that millions of children in poor countries throughout the world have died simply because nobody knew how to rehydrate them when they were suffering from diarrhoea. In Bangladesh with its annual floods, the chances of a child drinking dirty water and succumbing to this easily preventable death were very high.

BRAC used its extensive network of village and women's groups, of schools and classes to teach people about the problem and about how to tackle it. Ten years later 13 million households out of 15 million nationwide had learned to prepare oral rehydration solution. BRAC had empowered the women and the communities.

Deaths of children under 5 fell from over 200 per 1000 to about 80 per 1000 between 1990 and 2005.[1] It was so much better than the Sub-Saharan African figure of 137 for 2005; but still massively higher than the British figure of 6.[2]

This was a practical lesson in simple solutions and community organisation. It was a story that contrasted very sharply, as I think Mr Abed knew it would, with the technical analysis and complicated planning processes that I had heard about elsewhere. He was deliberately contrasting the simplicity of this self-help approach with the complex processes of international development.

BRAC is a remarkable organisation. Involving 100 000 staff and 70 000 volunteers it reaches out into all parts of Bangladesh and has, in recent years, spread its activities and philosophy to other countries.

It runs health clinics and education classes and works with women to help them understand their rights and improve their position in society. It has always focussed on the poorest people and those most excluded from the normal life and services of the country, but it also recognises that people need to aspire to the best and has, for example, created a BRAC University to provide wider opportunity for learning and development.

Its approach to empowering people is to help them improve their own lives and to make those improvements self-sustaining. As part of this approach it uses business methods to achieve its social goals. It helps women learn the skills to run small enterprises, supports them by providing small loans from the BRAC Bank, has created shops to help small enterprises sell their products and founded six farms to provide good-quality chicks to be grown on by small farmers. BRAC is a social enterprise that is a big business in its own right. BRAC Bank alone has 6 million borrowers and a turnover of US$4 billion.

BRAC's version of empowering people is to help them gain economic independence as well as have rights and a voice in their society.[3]

The key to our learning

BRAC illustrates many of the things that can be learned from poorer countries. These fall into three groups: firstly there are different ideas, attitudes and approaches to health and resources; secondly, there are specific innovations in policy or treatment; and thirdly, there is much that can be learned from working together. We start here with the first and most important of these.

In the last chapter we saw how it was the ideas, values and world view of western medicine and society that were imported so effectively into poor countries and which continue to influence them so powerfully in so many different ways today.

The most important thing that the rich can learn from the poor is, in precisely the same way, the different ideas, behaviours and attitudes that can help them conceive and conceptualise their world differently and find new solutions to new as well as old problems. They can learn to see the world differently and act differently.

Poorer countries simply don't have the critical mass of professionals, the scientists, the commercial activity and the governments' funding of healthcare, which are so essential to our understanding of western scientific medicine. That doesn't mean that progress can't be made, but rather that people have developed another set of ideas for dealing with the problems they face.

These ideas, which have been developed in different countries all over the world, can't replace those of western scientific medicine – we still need professionalism, science, commerce and government – but they can enhance and complement them and help them reach into areas they didn't previously reach.

We will briefly outline six of these ideas here, all of which relate to each other. We have already seen how BRAC has developed an approach that uses business methods to achieve social goals; that empowers people by helping them become economically independent and deals with health as part of peoples' lives and not as something completely separate.

We will see in a moment how leaders in Africa and Brazil have developed new ways of training and deploying health staff, in the absence of all those health professionals; brought public health and clinical medicine closer together and made the best use of whatever resources were to hand.

Combinations of these six are proving vital in many poorer countries.

Learning from the poor – a different set of ideas that can complement western scientific medicine

Figure 6.1 lists the key features that distinguish the approaches being adopted so successfully in many poorer countries. They combine a pragmatic common sense with vision and creativity. All the examples given over the next few pages use a combination of two or more of these approaches in the way they work.

- *Social enterprises use business methods to achieve social ends*

- *Empowering people means helping them become economically independent as well as having rights and a voice*

- *Health is dealt with as a part of people's lives and not as something completely separate*

- *Health workers are trained to meet local needs and not just for the professions*

- *Public health and clinical medicine are brought together*

- *Best use is made of the resources to hand*

Figure 6.1 A different set of ideas that can complement western scientific medicine

Bangladesh might seem an unlikely place from which to learn. It is a fascinating country, but it has appalling problems. Poor, it comes 147th out of 179 on the Human Development Index Ratings.[4] Overcrowded, with 153 million people in 144 thousand square kilometres, it is one of the ten most densely populated countries in the world and the only large country anywhere near the top of a list headed by Macau, Monaco, Singapore and Taiwan. Its traffic congestion, however, probably comfortably tops the world rankings.

A large part of Bangladesh floods each year, giving it the vital water and nutrients it needs for its crops. In a bad year, however, the run off of melting snow from the Himalayas and the monsoon of summer can turn a routine annual flood into catastrophe.

Following the great improvements in oral rehydration and similar successes on immunisation the biggest single killer of children is now drowning.

This is a country where government is weak and where a non-elected acting Chief Minister held power for the whole of 2008 because the politicians could not agree on arrangements for elections, let alone the distribution of power. There seems little prospect of them facing up to the problems that climate change may bring as seas rise around the low-lying country. Despite all this, Bangladesh has a very strong spirit of enterprise and community action and has produced some other remarkable social enterprises. Muhammad Yunus's Grameen Bank, the pioneer of microfinance and microcredit, has had enormous influence and impact internationally. There are now many large and small microfinance institutions around the world that are able to lend small sums of money to people, mainly women, to set up or run small enterprises and help them to save money for use later.

These enterprises are capable of having enormous impact. A World Bank study found that 40 percent of the entire reduction of poverty in rural Bangladesh was directly attributable to microfinance.[5] There is a long tradition of such schemes elsewhere in the world and there are now more than 3100 such institutions worldwide, which have 92 million clients, more than 80% of whom are women.[6]

There are many other smaller organisations in Bangladesh that embody the same spirit and this same social enterprise approach of using business methods to achieve social purposes. They appear to sit comfortably alongside other commercial organisations. I asked people in Bangladesh why there was this spirit of self-help and community entrepreneurship. They suggested it had grown out of their battle for independence from Pakistan when they had to rely only on their internal resources and their community solidarity. Wherever it comes from, it is very powerful and gives a sense of hope to a country facing such a difficult and uncertain future.

"A package of development services that they themselves decide on, design, implement and eventually finance"

BRAC is not the only such organisation and Bangladesh is not the only country where these developments have occurred. URVAL, 500 miles away in Rajasthan in India, had been established in 1986 to promote the economic and social development of remote communities in the Thar Desert. Established explicitly on Ghandian principles of self-determination, one of its early projects was the development of a cooperative amongst the weavers of the area.

More than 300 self-employed weavers, each working from a loom at their own home, had built an organisation that allowed them to share the purchasing of raw materials and the marketing, production planning and sales that kept them in business. Together they create many of the wonderful and bright cloths worn by Rajasthan women that are so characteristic of the region.

Arvind Ohja, a man of medium height in his 50s, with the beard common to all men in the area and wearing a long woollen waistcoat, woven locally, as an outer garment, was my guide to the organisation. He is intellectual and both passionate and eloquent about the organisation of which he was one of the original members. I asked him how he had become involved and, in a story with biblical overtones, he told me that he had been working in local government when he met the founder. Within an hour he had decided to join him and 15 years on, he has never looked back or regretted it.

URVAL expands into the areas where it is needed. Eye health was one. Eyes suffer in the dry, dusty and often windy conditions of the desert. URVAL went into partnership with Sightsavers International to run eye camps, bring treatment to remote areas and find ways to rehabilitate people who had become blind. Arvind took me to a single-story house made of concrete blocks miles from the nearest town and introduced me to Manohar Kanwar, who had been blind from childhood and lived with her mother and sister. Thanks to URVAL and Sightsavers she had learned to cook and look after herself and earned money sewing edging onto material prepared by the weavers.

The same themes that we saw in BRAC are evident here: social enterprise, economic empowerment and the treatment of health alongside other issues. URVAL, and Arvind himself, have a very powerful vision for what they are aiming to do: to lead the poor towards self-reliance by making available to them a package of development services that they themselves decide on, design, implement and eventually finance.

In Nicaragua another inspirational group, the Movimiento Comunal Nicaragüense (MCN), was created in 1978 to improve living conditions through social and community development, gender equality and environmental protection. They work in about half the country, mostly in rural areas, and have a presence in 120 municipalities and 2000 local communities. Like BRAC they are able to mobilise thousands of people, mostly women, such as community leaders, teachers and midwives to improve public health.

The group's efforts have led to advances in literacy, polio eradication and reduction of maternal and child mortality rates.[7,8] Most recently, MCN has centred its efforts on young people, aiming to improve gender relations, wipe out violence, prevent sexually transmitted infections (STI's) and reduce teen pregnancies.[9]

URVAL and MCN may be half a world apart, but both of these organisations are a world away from the usual professionalised models of development.

Training people for the job that needs doing

As we have seen in earlier chapters, there is a critical shortage of health workers in many countries and, as a result, there has been a great deal of effort put into finding ways to fill the gap. Over the next few pages we will move to Africa and Brazil as we explore some of the solutions people have found. All of them have in common that they are training people for the job that needs doing with reference, but not deference, to the established health professions.

I wasn't surprised to hear that BRAC had links with some of these developments in Africa. Colin McCord, a young American surgeon, worked at BRAC in the 1970s and subsequently moved to Mozambique, where he became involved in training non-medical staff to undertake obstetric surgery.

Mozambique, war torn and very poor, had very few doctors and an appalling health record. Thousands of mothers died in childbirth each year and thousands of babies and young children perished. In 1984 carefully selected health workers were recruited from various rural settings for a 2-year course to become tecnico de cirurgia and be able to undertake obstetric surgery.

These tecnicos de cirurgia in Mozambique might be called obstetric surgeons or clinical officers or medical officers or medical licentiates elsewhere in Africa. They are equivalent to what Europeans or Americans call surgically trained assistant medical officers. Development workers and academics tend to use the terminology 'mid-level workers' in order to distinguish them from much lower skilled community health workers and from the traditionally educated health professionals such as doctors, nurses and midwives.

These tecnicos have over the years become the mainstay of the country's obstetric service in rural areas. A study published in 2007 showed that 92% of caesarean sections, obstetric hysterectomies and laparotomies for ectopic pregnancies performed in all district hospitals in the country during the course of a year were carried out by tecnicos de cirurgia.[10]

A second study also published in 2007 tells a remarkable story about how the training and employment of tecnicos is having an impact on the perennial problem of retaining skilled health workers in rural areas. It showed that 88% of tecnicos de cirurgia from the three graduating classes surveyed were still working in rural areas 7 years after graduation. None of the doctors, by contrast, from the same 3 years were working in rural areas 7 years after graduation.[11]

Earlier studies had shown that there were no clinically significant differences in postoperative outcomes between surgeries undertaken by tecnicos and by doctors and that postoperative mortality rates for 10 258 patients operated on by tecnicos were very low at 0.4% for emergency surgery and 0.1% for elective.[12,13] In laypeople's terms: the work was done as well as doctors would have done it – if there had been any. These and similar experiences elsewhere in the world have inspired the establishment of the Health Systems Strengthening for Equity Programme, which, through research and advocacy, is seeking to build a research base and strengthen support for mid-level providers to be used more extensively.

It is precisely the sort of programme that is needed to ensure that the world learns about these developments and is encouraged to give them a higher priority.

This one is a deserter!

This extraordinary success story is mirrored elsewhere in Africa.

I visited the District Hospital in Jinja in Uganda on behalf of Sightsavers in 2008 and met some of the students being trained there as ophthalmology assistants. At the end of the year they would be able to assess their patients and do a range of operations including ones for trachoma, that awful disease of the eyelids that causes great pain and leads to blindness. After 1 year's further experience they could return to Jinja for further training with the eventual prospect of becoming cataract surgeons.

I talked with 12 bright, young people in their classroom: a concrete block built single-story building no different from thousands of other schoolrooms in Africa. Their learning aids were a single overhead projector and, most important of all, access to the nearby eye ward where their teacher, Dr Bantu, operated.

I asked them about themselves and their hopes and fears for the course. They were highschool graduates who had all done 1 year of some health-related work before coming on the course. They were proud to be there and looking forward to a future working in their home districts. They laughed and joked with each other as they talked about going home and taking up a job with the responsibility for looking after the eye health needs of a local population. It was obviously both exciting and nerve-racking at the same time. These young people were going to carry a lot of responsibility.

Sightsavers, as is our normal practice, had set up the course in collaboration with the Government and, whilst we paid for the training, the Government guaranteed the students subsequent employment, provided they passed their exams. Dr Bantu, who is a middle-aged man of Asian ancestry approaching retirement, sees his role very explicitly as providing trained health workers to meet the needs of his country and he is therefore very interested in what becomes of his pupils after they leave him.

He showed me a register with the names of all the students who had graduated from his class over its 12-year existence. Going through them one by one, he told me where they were now. He was proud that he had at least one graduate working in each District of the country, even the north, which was still very troubled and, in some parts almost a war zone. Several had gone on to be cataract surgeons and one, to his great pride, had successfully trained to become a fully qualified ophthalmic surgeon.

Sadly 12 of the 100 or so graduates were already dead, reflecting the AIDS epidemic in his country. One he had lost touch with and one, to his horror, was working in the private sector in the capital Kampala. "This one", he said jabbing at the name on the page with disgust, "is a deserter!"

Whilst the group I met were on a 1-year course to become ophthalmology assistants, others were trained as cataract surgeons. These surgeons have become the backbone and mainstay of cataract surgery in large parts of East and West Africa. As with the tecnicos, the cataract surgeons have very good complication rates.

The moment when a person's sight is restored is a remarkable thing to witness. I met two of Dr Bantu's patients as their bandages were being taken off after a cataract operation. The first, an elderly man, remained impassive for a long instant as if nothing were different, before the beginnings of a smile appeared on his face. "What do you see?" he was asked. "Muzungu", he replied: a white man!

The second was a middle-aged woman who reacted immediately when the bandages were removed. Beaming, she stood up from the bed and began a shuffling dance, swaying her large hips and ululating her pleasure. "What are you going to do now that you can see?" someone asked. "Find a new husband!" she replied. I wondered why all the men had fled laughing as I innocently stood my ground and waited for the translation.

Planning with the resources you have

Another man who is very explicit about the need to make the best use of what is available is the Minister of Health for Ethiopia, Dr Tedros Adhanom Ghebreyesus. He is responsible for health in one of the fastest growing and poorest countries in Africa, where the annual expenditure on health is US$22 per person and the population now exceeds 80 million.[14]

His whole health plan is based on the premise that you train and employ the people you need to deal with the tasks that need doing. The foundation of the Ethiopian service is a very large number of health extension workers who work locally and are primarily concerned with health promotion but carry out some treatment programmes. Above them sit the mid-level workers: the emergency surgeons, direct entry anaesthetists, general clinical officers and others who carry out the bulk of the direct patient work. Above them are the doctors and nurses and other clinical professionals and scientists.[15]

Dr Tedros's view is straightforward: 80% of the burden of disease in Ethiopia is due to communicable diseases, and most cases can be prevented or treated by community and mid-level workers. We must use the assets at hand and provide what we can to our communities. There is no justification for the shortages of community and mid-level workers.[16] All groups of health workers are needed. Ethiopia and Mozambique – described earlier – need the highest educated scientists and doctors as well as health extension workers. The fundamental questions are about the proportions of the different types of health workers, the relationships between them and, of course, how easy it is to get them.

Brazil can also tell an impressive story. Since the 1980s Brazil has pursued a policy of training family health teams to provide local care for the country's entire far-flung population, many of whom have to travel for days to reach a hospital. Each team consists of a doctor, a nurse and up to six nursing auxiliaries. As many as 25 000 teams were created by 2007 and covered over 60% of the population. One of the central aspects of this development has been the upgrading of the skills of existing auxiliary nurses, taking them into new areas of expertise and skill where they, like the health extension workers, deal with health promotion as well as treatment.[17]

Community health workers – linking public health and clinical medicine

The earlier discussion has concentrated on the so-called mid-level workers, people who have received the substantial amount of training needed to perform caesarean sections or cataract surgery, and on auxiliary nurses, who are an integral part of a local health team and a local health system. They are all part of a formal health team.

There is also, however, a very strong emphasis on community in the provision of healthcare and the promotion of health in many poor countries. This goes far beyond the notion of a formal health service. There is no simple picture here and a spectrum of activity from government-initiated schemes to local developments and groups concerned with advocacy and education.

Pakistan's Lady Health Workers Programme is an enormous enterprise that was started in 2005 by the Government with the aim of deploying 100 000 workers across the country to help improve health at the village level. Each worker is a resident of the community she serves and is attached to a government health facility from which she receives training, a small allowance and medical supplies.

India has similar programmes and I met two of India's thousands of Accredited Social Health Workers (ASHAs) in a small brick-built hut in a village 50 miles south of Kolkata in Western Bengal. These ASHAs have been recruited across India to provide advice and information for their neighbours, to promote immunisation and contraception and to track pregnancies, antenatal care and health issues.

The two women showed me proudly the various handwritten charts and tables they kept that recorded the names of the whole population, identified who was pregnant, who was using contraception and whose children had been immunised. In the gloom of early evening, with no electricity and no lamps, they talked proudly about their work and how they kept an eye on the old people in the village as well as on water levels and how they reported it all to the local authorities.

My western eyes noted that there was no attempt to preserve patient confidentiality. I was reminded of the discussions in the UK about who could have access to patient and public records and how this had become more complicated by the existence of electronic records that with a keystroke, intentional or otherwise, could be sent around the world. This was one problem they didn't yet face in western Bengal, although with India's IT industry it might only be a matter of months away.

The theme of health, not illness, pervades the work of community health workers in Africa. Dr Brian Chituwo, formerly Minister of Health in Zambia, himself a clinician – an orthopaedic surgeon trained in London – goes further. He sees them in his country as promoting health, a healthy life and a healthy community; they are a core part of the development and future prosperity of his country.

Minister Tedros in Ethiopia is also very keen to point out that the most local level of his health system is made up of Health Extension Workers whose primary role is promotion of health and prevention of diseases. They do give some treatment, but, as he always stresses, this is secondary. He wants to create a service founded on health, not disease.

There is a deliberate intention to bring together public health and clinical medicine to the benefit of both. Ghana's 2006 health plan went even further and was based one the idea of involving the whole community and using all its knowledge and energy in laying the foundation for future health. It is one of several that seek to involve the traditional healers, reasoning that they are an extra resource which, engaged in the right way, can help provide information and support the work of the trained health workers. This can be a risky practice, unless healers can be persuaded to forgo many of their traditional practices.

Researchers for a survey on blindness in Nigeria in 2008, for example, found that traditional healers had treated many people with cataracts by 'couching'.[18] This is an old and barbaric practice, mentioned by Pliny, where the clouded lens is knocked off the front of the eye with a wooden implement, thereby allowing light but not focussed sight to reach the retina at the back. It offers a semblance of improvement with the patient able to distinguish day from night, but does so much damage to the eye that only rarely can a new artificial lens be fitted and sight restored.

Communities can also play a very important role in getting health messages through to individuals and stopping these dangerous practices. I met a group of villagers in Uganda who worked with Sightsavers to take messages about eye health to their own and neighbouring communities. They did it through the African media of play acting and music.

Eight of them played out a scene for me in front of the village's one-roomed clinic. It was a straightforward tale full of drama and humour. A woman with a pain in her eye went to a traditional healer, who gave her a potion to rub in. It made it much worse. She sobbed with pain as she went completely blind. A wise neighbour intervened and took her to the nurse in the clinic. In due course her eyesight returned and all was well. It was simply done but very effective.

On the other hand, traditional birth attendants are frequently involved in care for pregnant women in many countries. Whilst they have skills very different from Mozambique's highly technically trained mid-level workers, they can bring experience, wisdom and care as part of a balanced team. In a striking reversal of previous official policy on the continent the African Union declared a Decade of Traditional Medicine starting in 2001 and has since adopted a policy for developing its use and integrating it into both policy and practice by 2010.[19]

These snapshots from different countries illustrate something of the range and scope of community health work. There continues, however, to be much debate and controversy over whether and to what extent these types of community workers are effective in keeping populations healthy. The evidence is becoming much clearer as researchers bring together the findings from several studies.

Community health workers can improve health outcomes through health promotion and deliver a range of treatments, which include vaccinations, malaria treatment, case management of childhood illness and adherence to treatment regimes. Research has shown that community health workers can contribute to reductions in child mortality[20-22] and specifically that the Pakistan Lady Health Worker programme has led to more women using antenatal care, having assistance at birth and using family planning services.[23]

The evidence also shows that these community worker programmes are most effective where they are integrated into the wider health system, they can refer on to more trained health workers and they have the opportunity for refresher or further training and supervision.[16] Many community worker programmes have failed for lack of these features. One of the reasons that China's famous 'bare foot doctors' were not in the end as successful as they might have been was that they were largely left to their own devices after their initial training, with no supervision and refresher or follow-up training. In these circumstances knowledge can decay and bad habits become ingrained. The remnants of the service, established in 1968 did survive into the 1990s, when wholesale privatisation of health services swept them away, with many setting up as individual private practitioners.[24]

Innovations in policy and treatment

These earlier examples have described the way people in poorer countries have developed different ways of looking at the world, challenging some of the western world's basic assumptions about traditional medicine, professionalism and government responsibilities. There is much to learn from their whole approach.

There are also examples of specific policies and practices that the West can learn from. Here we identify just a few from the many there are.

The first one is a major area of policy that may have very significant long-term effects. In the 1990's the Mexican Ministry of Health had recognised that the poorest people in the population often didn't have the education or motivation to adopt healthy practices, so started giving people specific payments as an incentive to change their behaviour and, for example, get a medical checkup for their children, attend antenatal clinics or enrol their children in school. This was so successful that Mexico has subsequently tied most of its social welfare programme to these sorts of actions and behaviour changes. In 2002 they set up Oportunidades as, in the language now used, a Conditional Cash Transfer programme designed to reach all parts of the population.

In 2004 Julio Frenk, the very innovative health minister of the time and now Dean of the School of Public Health at Harvard, took this further by establishing a programme of health insurance for the poor called Seguro Popular. His aim, as he described in a Lancet article was to achieve "universal access to high-quality services with social protection for all". Both the Oportunidades and Seguro Popular have been very influential globally - in richer and poorer countries.[25]

Many countries in Latin America, Asia and Africa now have similar programmes and in 2007 Mayor Bloomberg of New York City set up the US$50 million Opportunity NYC programme and acknowledged that it was based on what he had learned from Mexico. In New York, too, there were problems with education and motivation and reaching those people most in need.

Another very significant example is the change that has been made in the way that AIDS treatment is administered globally. I recall listening to Professor Michel Kazatchkine, the Director of the Global Fund, talking at a seminar at Imperial College in London about how worldwide treatment of AIDS had been influenced by what was learned in Africa.

One of his examples stood out for me. African patients, he observed, were not as accustomed as people in Europe and North America to attend follow-up clinics. It was therefore necessary to find ways to give as much treatment as possible on each occasion, changing drug regimes as required. It was quickly recognised that this would be useful elsewhere and these methods of delivering treatments learned in Africa are now the standard protocols worldwide.

Other examples come from westerners working in poorer countries, where the resources they would normally use simply aren't available and they have had to be creative. Steve Mannion, who works part of the year in Newcastle in the UK and part in Malawi, is an orthopaedic surgeon who has changed the way club-foot in newborn children is treated as a result of his experience in Malawi.

The practice in rich countries had been in recent years to carry out a lengthy and difficult operation to re-align and straighten the foot. Faced with a vast number of patients in Malawi needing treatment, Steve cast around for other ways of helping them and came across an old technique invented by an Italian and based on repeated manipulations. In simple terms, the foot is bent as far as possible into the right position each week and bound in place. After several weeks of such treatment, the condition has all but disappeared. This is now the standard treatment in London, Paris and New York as well as Lilongwe and Blantyre.

Others come from local people addressing local issues. Aravind Eye Care in southern India was faced with enormous numbers of patients needing cataract surgery and simply could not afford the expensive materials and techniques then in use in rich countries. They set out to develop new methodologies and materials.[26] They succeeded. Their intraocular lens, costing around US$2 apiece, is now used in 120 countries around the world; whilst their operational and other research operates at world standards.

Professor Alan Rosen, a Psychiatric and Public Health specialist from the Universities of Sydney and Wollongong, has written about comparative studies by the World Health Organization (WHO), which have demonstrated better long-term outcome for schizophrenia in developing countries. He reports that "*These findings still generate some professional contention and disbelief, as they challenge outdated assumptions that people generally do not recover from schizophrenia and that the outcomes of western treatments and rehabilitation must be superior. However, these results have proven to be remarkably robust, on the basis of international replications and 15–25-year follow-up studies. Explanations for this phenomenon are still at the hypothesis level, but include: (1) greater inclusion or retained social integration in the community in developing countries, so that the person maintains a role or status in the society; (2) involvement in traditional healing rituals, reaffirming communal inclusion and solidarity; (3) availability of a valued work role that can be adapted to a lower level of functioning; (4) availability of an extended kinship or communal network, so that family tension and burden are diffused, and there is often low negatively 'expressed emotion' in the family.*"[27]

I have quoted Professor Rosen at some length because his account deals with scepticism of his colleagues and suggests some of the reasons why the treatment is so successful. It has potential for changing the way schizophrenia is managed in richer countries.

I have found many Americans and Britons who, when asked about learning from their experiences in poorer countries, immediately give me examples. Professor Philippa Easterbrook of London University sent me a long list based on her experiences in working at the Infectious Diseases Institute in Uganda. It included the exploring of different models of delivery of care, innovative approaches to scaling up of counselling and testing through the use of family members and the community, the involvement of people living with HIV as agents of change and a more holistic approach to care. She also remarked on the recognition of the central role of spirituality, as well as music in the delivery of care in Africa, and on the adoption of 'task sharing or shifting' with leading roles for nurses and pharmacists in delivery of Anti-Retroviral Therapy. All of these potentially have application elsewhere.

Figure 6.2 lists some of the specific policies and practices developed in poorer countries that have much wider relevance.

New policy, practices and products:

- *Conditional cash transfers – to incentivise healthy behaviour*

- *Changing drug-giving protocols – where patients rarely attend outpatient clinics and are hard to track*

- *New and better standard treatment for club-foot – where there weren't the resources for the old approach*

- *New lens and protocols – where the old ones were too expensive*

- *Better long-term outcomes for schizophrenia – through inclusion and community involvement*

Figure 6.2 Some specific innovations from poorer countries

These few accounts illustrate people using the resources they have and finding ways around local obstacles to the delivery of healthcare. There are many more like them. There is nothing, however, very unusual about learning from poorer countries when we turn to experience in the wider context of commercial development.

In health we see that a number of countries, including Thailand, Singapore and India, have developed new ways of providing private health services for 'health tourists' and are challenging the long-established providers of the USA and Europe on both quality and cost. In other areas of business leading organisations and thinkers are setting out explicitly to learn from what is happening in poorer countries.[28]

Practice is changing in richer countries as well

Richer countries also have problems in staffing their services; this is in part due to shortages but it is also due to costs, with the employment of health workers making up more than half the total cost of services. As a result there has been a great deal of experimentation and innovation there as well.

There are, for example, now many physicians' assistants in the USA who are taking on work that in other circumstances was previously only done by physicians, whilst nurses in the UK have extended their role in many directions to include, for example, undertaking endoscopies and prescribing drugs within a limited set of indications and a restricted formulary. There are now many different sorts of aides and technical assistants.

How, one might reasonably ask, is what is happening in poor countries any different from this? What can be learned from poor countries?

The biggest difference is whether these developments are absolutely central or not to the health system. The tecnicos de cirurgia do the bulk of the work in rural Mozambique. Clinical officers in other parts of Africa do a great deal of the day-to-day clinical work. Perhaps even more importantly, the planners and policymakers see their contribution as central to their thinking and plans.

In rich countries these developments are generally still seen as peripheral; they are typically fitted in around the main business, which remains firmly the preserve of the professions. Even where, as in my own country, the UK, we increased the numbers of trained but unqualified staff, we continued to increase the number of professionally trained staff.

It is a very similar story when we look at community organisations and action in richer countries. There are many social enterprise pioneers in richer countries as well. There are more than 300 groups in the UK in membership of CAN, the social enterprise network. It was co-founded by Lord Andrew Mawson, who over 25 years has also developed a group of linked social enterprises in East London that offer housing, education, health and social services to local people through the work of the Bromley-by-Bow Centre.

His work has many parallels with that of Fazle Hassan Abed with BRAC in Bangladesh; except that he is not part of the mainstream of public activity in the way that Mr Abed is. In writing up his own story about the achievements and frustrations of the last 25 years in developing these programmes, Andrew describes how he has very often found it difficult to be taken seriously by the authorities, despite the growing scale and obvious success of most of his ventures. This difficulty continues today. He, I and others are currently working with government officials in the UK to try to find ways to link the bottom-up approaches of social enterprise organisations with the, necessarily, top-down approaches of government and public authorities. There is potentially enormous benefit from combining the power of both approaches, but we have not yet found a way of doing so in our society.[29]

In countries like Bangladesh, with little public or state provision, these organisations become the mainstream. In countries like the UK they are very often peripheral and, whilst they may be doing very good work, are treated as such.

Health continues to be a professional preserve.

However, the world is changing. There are many more such developments in rich countries and the balance of numbers and activity is beginning, still largely unnoticed, to shift. The changes in staffing structures will undoubtedly accelerate as cost pressures bite and health planners recognise more clearly that they don't need to see the world through the framework of the traditional professions.

Money will make the world turn upside down

We may not, as yet, have noticed that the world is shifting. Eventually, however, I suspect that it will be costs that will force us all to understand how policies in rich countries have to change. Norway, as described in Chapter 4, has undertaken a study that showed that staffing would need to increase massively, perhaps by 30%, simply due to the ageing of its population.

It has considered in detail how, if it has to recruit workers from aboard to deal with this shortfall, it might compensate other countries for the costs of training and the loss of skilled health workers.[30] I asked the Noregian Minister and senior officials in early 2009 whether they had given similar consideration to reducing their reliance on highly educated professional staff. They didn't feel it was necessary or appropriate to do so.

Norway has substantial oil revenues, a small population and a sovereign wealth fund and may not have to face up to this difficult change. There is no reason, however, to think that the UK or the USA or France or Germany can avoid the issue. Somewhere, sometime, explicitly or by stealth, politicians and health planners will have to alter this over-reliance on highly paid professionals and start to introduce many more health workers trained to do the tasks that need doing. They will have to alter the balance of their workforce and do what the Africans and South Americans are doing today.

The simple pyramids in Figure 6.3 compare the workforces in Ethiopia and the UK and illustrate the differences.

Both systems are 'bottom up' in structure. Only things that can't be handled by the health extension workers are pushed up this pyramid and so on through each level in turn. The biggest difference is in the proportion of people employed at each level of the pyramid. In Ethiopia the biggest preponderance of people are in the lower parts; England and other richer countries are much more top heavy. They have a flat topped pyramid.

This key difference means that in rich countries, whatever the structure of their service and its intended operation, the whole dynamic, as we saw in Chapter 3, is to pull more and more activity through to the highest and most specialised level. In countries such as

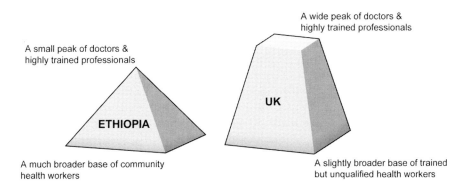

The different pyramids in Ethiopia and the UK

A small peak of doctors &
highly trained professionals

A wide peak of doctors &
highly trained professionals

ETHIOPIA

UK

A much broader base of community
health workers

A slightly broader base of trained
but unqualified health workers

the UK pyramid is 40 x larger than the Ethiopian one

Figure 6.3 The different workforce distribution in Ethiopia and the UK

the USA, or in France until this year, where patients can directly refer themselves to specialists, this is even more pronounced. The result is the expensive and wasteful top-down hospital-based and highly specialised services that are so familiar in rich countries.

We will undoubtedly see a similar trend in Ethiopia and other countries as people aim for greater things. The world doesn't stand still and the thousands of people who are mid-level workers today will aspire to be nurses and doctors tomorrow. Minister Tedros and his successors will have difficulty in keeping the appropriate proportions between the levels of staff in his service. The skill mix will become richer with greater numbers of qualified people, each of them with a reasonable expectation that their skills will be rewarded with higher levels both of pay and responsibility.

Costs and qualifications go hand in hand from the length of training to the cost of employment. In Mozambique an economic evaluation of the comparative performance of tecnicos and doctors in 2007 showed that the costs per major obstetric procedure for tecnicos de cirurgia average about one-third of physician costs over their careers. The costs of training and deploying tecnicos de cirurgia is less than one-quarter that of physician specialists.[10] The figures will be different but the pattern similar in other countries.

Political will and the art of the possible

Making change of this sort will be difficult, both for good reasons and for bad. The good reasons are concerns about whether patients will actually see the highly trained specialist when they need to or whether they will see a less-trained person who will miss the vital information and fail to make the right diagnosis. This is a real concern and can only be dealt with by making sure that the less-trained person always has access to the higher trained and knows how to refer and is listened to when they do. This isn't easy to do. It requires sufficient numbers of staff at both levels as well as good training and good systems.

The bad reasons are about protectionism and about professions and trade unions wanting to hang on to jobs and to territory.

These types of arguments have been conducted in international development circles for years with controversy about whether or not community health workers in particular served a useful purpose. For the time being the evidence described earlier in this chapter seems to have convinced the sceptics and there is a lot of support for the sorts of development described in Ethiopia and for so-called 'task shifting', described by the WHO as a process of delegation whereby tasks are moved to less specialised health workers.[31]

These battles are still to be fought in richer countries. Experience to date shows that they have not yet really started.

The Brazilian plan, its *Family Health Program*, has been sustained for 20 years and during the tenure of successive presidents and governments. This is a remarkable demonstration of the sustained and consistent political commitment that is the first and most important criterion for success in any major change in a health system.

It is interesting to note that the successive Brazilian governments have steered a careful path between taking a radical approach to the training and employment of health workers whilst at the same time maintaining the position and status of the traditional health professionals. The new auxiliary nurses are in many cases people who were already undertaking some kind of health role in an unsupervised and unregulated fashion in the country. Their training by government brought them within a regulated system. This has created a very welcome improvement in the quality and continuity of care. It has also meant, however, that the new auxiliary nurses did not threaten the power and position of the professionals. In some ways they reinforced the status quo.

The fact that the status quo hasn't changed was well illustrated for me at a meeting I was at in Africa where the Brazilian Deputy Minister took and made a succession of slightly agitated phone calls. He told me that the doctors in Brazil were threatening to go on strike because a minister had suggested that nurses might take on a task reserved for doctors.

Brazil is one of those countries with a very restricted list of roles and tasks that can be done by professionals other than doctors. Nurses are far more limited in what they can do than in Europe or North America. This demarcation is enforced by law. The doctors' unions were clearly not ready for any task shifting. The Government was not prepared for a fight on that occasion and later that day Deputy Minister told me it had backed down.

We can tell a story with some similarities in recent years in the UK. In 2000 the Government set out a 10-year programme, The NHS Plan, to deliver radical improvements in the quality and performance of the NHS in England. The Government's steady will and consistency over the years has, undoubtedly, helped to bring about real improvement. However, we, I was the NHS Chief Executive at the time, also worked carefully to try to bring as many as possible of the traditionally powerful groups with us on the journey.

The Plan set targets to increase the number of doctors employed in the NHS by 10 000 and the number of nurses by 30 000. Both targets were achieved, with at least 20 000 doctors and 60 000 nurses being employed by 2005. Over the same period, although there was no target, around 70 000 other people were employed in direct patient care. Some of these were in traditional nursing assistant-type roles, but many were in new roles of imaging technicians, physiotherapy assistants and mental health counsellors.

This big change in practice was quietly managed and was not really registered as the significant change in policy that it was.[32] However, it was hidden by the fact that we had increased the numbers of highly trained professionals at the same time. In retrospect I wonder, if radical as we were in so many other areas, we missed the opportunity to change the conventional mindset about education, training and the roles of health workers. It is an issue my successors have to face up to as our population ages and our finances dictate.

With this in mind we need to be careful that we don't see 'task shifting' in developing countries as a purely temporary expedient and only necessary until enough staff and money is available. It is equally important that we don't overcomplicate and overmedicalise things that are, in truth, quite simple and concerned more with the emotions than with science and professionalism.

Perhaps most importantly of all, we need to make sure that we don't think that quality only refers to clinical quality and outcomes or that only highly trained professionals can deliver high-quality care. It depends on what the patient needs.

Partnerships

There is a long tradition of partnerships between hospitals, universities and other organisations in rich and poor countries. At the same time many individuals have found their own way to work in poorer countries as volunteers or temporary members of staff. Over the last few years more and more students have gone to spend periods of time working abroad. There is an increasing amount of interchange in person and over the Internet and phone networks.

At their best these partnerships between institutions in different countries can be very effective. They can have enormous impact if they are based on the needs of the poorer country and built up through long-term relationships of respect. At their worst, when they are short term and badly thought through and executed, they can lead to wasted effort by both parties and to people being badly bruised by the experience.

I have been shown or told about many examples in Africa and India of equipment sent out from the UK that was not suitable, required parts, maintenance and even power that wasn't available locally and had just been left to rot. I was also told of people flying in to help who did so briefly and then left, having disrupted the hospital for the period of their residence. If people are coming to help, I was told frequently, they need to stay for a longer period or come back regularly to work, train people locally and share their experience and expertise.

There are about 100 UK organisations that have long-term partnerships with others abroad and many more from all over Europe and North America. They are mainly grouped around the Tropical Health Education Trust (THET), which has developed approaches to good practice and now runs a UK Government grant scheme to promote such partnerships.[33]

Brazil has built up strong links with the six Portuguese-speaking countries in Africa and shares a development network with them. Whilst each arrangement is individual, many of these partnerships work on the basis of teams from the richer country going to work for a period in the poorer one, offering training and expertise. This may be followed by people from the poorer country coming back to the richer one for further training and experience with the whole programme and exchanges being dictated by the needs of the poorer country.

There are other health partnerships in other countries. MEMISA is a network of Belgian organisations supporting health programmes in Asia, Africa and Latin America.[34] The ESTHER project in France involves 55 health partnerships between French hospitals and their counterparts in 15 countries in Asia and Africa.[35]

Some of the gains for the poorer country are obvious such as having skilled people, albeit for a limited but regular period, who can do particular tasks and can train locals. Sometimes these visits have led to new services being developed with continuing support provided by email and phone. The partnerships also provide a more hidden benefit by offering professional support to the, often isolated, clinical and other staff in the poorer country. I have heard people talk of the importance of not being alone and of feeling part of their wider profession and involved in global events.

The gains for the richer country can also be considerable. Part of this is about people seeing the world differently and understanding that things can be done differently. They develop greater flexibility and adaptability. It is interesting to hear from UK doctors who have worked in Africa or Asia, about how when they were faced with enormous numbers of patients and little in the way of equipment or drugs, they have been forced to improvise and invent ways to help them. Many have found this greatly exhilarating. Free of protocols, procedures and policies they have had to rely on their own resources and behave, as one radiologist friend told me, "like a proper doctor".

In the best cases they have been able to bring something of their experiences and ideas back to the UK. This is not always true, of course; some UK doctors have hated the experience and found that they were not suited to this sort of medicine. Others, however, seem to look back on their time abroad, even if it were only for a short 6-week medical student elective, as one of the most formative of their life.

There is an odd echo here of the way I have heard leading African doctors talk about their time in medical studies in the UK. Two ministers have told me separately that each time they come to London they pay their respects at their Alma Mater. Something of the same sentiment and affection appears to attach to a British doctor's time spent early in their career in Africa or Asia.

For the UK and other countries with large numbers of recent immigrants this sharing of experience between different countries and traditions can be very important for another very practical reason. Knowledge of their culture, tradition and practices is enormously useful to the clinician in London faced with patients from halfway round the world.

This is the basis of many international collaborations such as the *North2north Partnership* between the North West Frontier Province in Pakistan and the North West and Yorkshire and Humberside Health Authorities in the UK. Many families from this area of

Pakistan have migrated over the years to the industrial towns of the north of England and planners and clinicians regularly share learning and experiences across 6000 miles.

There are also shared benefits in research and education with collaboration based on learning from the diseases and conditions so prevalent in poor countries but which may threaten other populations as well. Figure 6.4 illustrates the benefits to both parties.

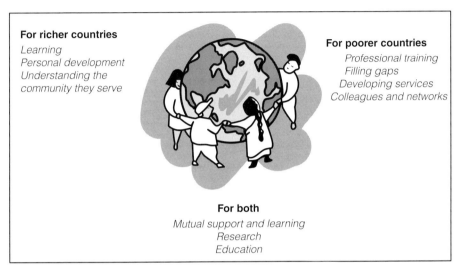

Figure 6.4 Gains from give and take in global health partnerships

I have described partnerships here as if the only ones involved two parties, one from a richer country and one from a poorer. There are many combinations, with advantages to be drawn from partnerships involving many parties and ones linking countries with the same needs, rich or poor. There are no boundaries to the arrangements that can be developed.

Given the desperate need to train more health workers in poorer countries, which we saw in Chapter 4, there is surely an opportunity here to build on this goodwill and expertise of health workers in richer countries. There is now a great deal of experience through these partnerships, but they remain very small in scale and barely impact on the problem.

Some donor governments are beginning to see this possibility and are supporting some of this partnership work and others see its importance for their own health services, but there is much potential that is as yet unrealised.

Conclusions

The chapter, written about what richer countries can learn from poorer ones, has also demonstrated how much poorer countries can and do learn from each other. Between them they are creating a new set of ideas that grow out of their own circumstances and experiences.

There are so many examples to choose from that I could have called it 1001 things that make a difference, but don't fit the paradigm. We have touched on a few examples here:

- Aravind Eye Hospital has very deliberately set out an approach to providing eye health services for poor populations.
- The policy of conditional cash transfers is being copied around the world.
- Señora Marcia Bassit, Brazil's Vice-Minister of Health, describing their progress in developing health workers at the first Global Health Workforce Alliance Forum in Kampala in 2008 was one of the stars of the conference. African health leaders, in particular, could see how the Brazilian model could apply in their countries.
- BRAC has set up programmes to export its methodologies in Africa as well as in the USA.

In many ways the biggest learning is about training people for the task that needs doing and not just for the professions. This is not new. My father-in-law, David Jenkins, who was referred to in the first chapter, reminded me that during World War II the British and French had both trained 'field surgeons' in the same way. In Africa, they did the same during the internal conflicts in Ethiopia and Mozambique much more recently.

Meanwhile the full potential of microfinance has not yet been realised. Some existing microfinance organisations already offer wider services and are likely to expand their activities much more extensively into health- and education-related matters – helping people both to improve their health and to cover the effects of what would otherwise be catastrophic illness.

Sheila Leatherman, a Professor from the University of North Carolina who researches and writes on this area, argues strongly that: "microfinance institutions can provide health education, motivation to change health practices, and referrals to good-quality health services, along with credit that stimulates increases in income and assets, while reducing people's vulnerability to financial and health crises."[36]

This chapter has also suggested that richer countries can learn from the ideas and approaches being generated in poorer ones. It has explored some of the very biggest themes in health that are of relevance to every country. There is the importance of empowering women, economically as well as politically. There is social enterprise and the bringing together of public health and clinical medicine. There is the freedom of thought needed to be able to plan training and education on the basis of what the country needs and not what the professions have decreed – a factor that will become more important as populations age and costs bite. There is the understanding of power and the necessity, for good or ill, of political involvement, determination and will.

There is, overwhelmingly, a sense of working with and through communities, villages and families and of generating energy to enable people themselves to make change and improve their lives. There is an understanding that health relates to everything else and an absence of rigid boundaries between actions to improve health and those to improve the economy or the environment.

These are all themes that we can find in rich countries as well as poor. However, they are not as prominent or as central and they are not yet by any means part of established knowledge and the mainstream of practice in rich countries. They are not yet fully part of the canon of knowledge and learning and don't yet take their place alongside science, commerce, professionalism and service. In rich countries we are, in many cases, failing to notice how the world, even in our own countries, is changing around us.

This chapter has also started to draw out the creativity inherent in bringing together all the different ways of looking at the world: bringing together different ideas, different experiences and different views. The freedom of movement and communication in the world, the great benefits of globalisation, allow us for the first time to mix, meld and merge as well as differentiate, choose and compare: to connect and to understand difference.

This blend is what, in the next chapter, I call 'new knowledge for the twenty-first century'.

References

1. World Health Organization. *Bangladesh Child Health Profile, 2007*. Available at: www.who.int/child_adolescent_health/data/media/cah_chp_bangladesh.pdf.
2. Verdier-Chouchane A. Combating under 5 mortality in Africa. *Policy Insights, OECD Development Centre* [Online] 2008; **65**. Available at: www.oecd.org/dataoecd/54/39/40583784.pdf.
3. Chen MA. *A Quiet Revolution: Women in transition in rural Bangladesh*. Dhaka: Brac Prokashana, 1983.
4. *Human Development Indices: A statistical update 2008 – HDI rankings*. Available at: hdr.undp.org/en/statistics/. [Accessed 15 September 2009].
5. Khandker S. Micro-finance and poverty: Evidence using panel data from Bangladesh. *World Bank Economic Review* 2005;**19**: 263–86.
6. Dunford C, Watson A. *From Microfinance to Macro Change: Integrating health education and microfinance to empower women and reduce poverty*. United Nations Population Fund, 2006. Available at: www.unfpa.org/upload/lib_pub_file/530_filename_advocacy.pdf.
7. United Nations. Egyptian doctor, Nicaraguan NGO receives top honours from UN. *UN News Centre*. [Online] 24 February 2009. Available at: www.un.org/apps/news/story.asp?NewsID=29999&Cr=population&Cr1=unfpa. [Accessed 25 September 2009].
8. Movimiento Comunal Nicaragüense. Available at: agora.ya.com/fcocca/nicar/. [Accessed 25 September 2009].
9. Ban presents UN population award to Egyptian doctor and Nicaraguan NGO. *UN News Centre*. [Online] 1 June 2009. www.un.org/apps/news/story.asp?NewsID=30989&Cr=unfpa&Cr1=. [Accessed 25 September 2009].
10. Kruk ME, Pereira C, Vaz F, Bergström S, Galea S. Economic evaluation of surgically trained assistant medical officers in performing major obstetric surgery in Mozambique. *Br J Obstet Gynaecol* 2007; **114**: 1253–60.
11. Pereira C, Cumbi A, Malalane R, Vaz F, McCord C, Bacci A, Bergström S. Meeting the need for emergency obstetrical care in Mozambique: work performance and history of medical doctors and assistant medical officers trained for surgery. *Br J Obstet Gynaecol* 2007; **114**: 1253–60.
12. Pereira C, Bugalho A, Bergström S, Vaz F, Cotiro M.A comparative study of caesarean deliveries by assistant medical officers and obstetricians in Mozambique. *Br J Obstet Gynaecol* 1996; **103**: 508–12.
13. Vaz F, Bergström S, Vaz ML, Langa J, Bughalo A. Training medical assistants for surgery. *Bull World Health Organ* 1999; **77**: 688–91.
14. World Health Organization. *Ethiopia country profile*. 2009. Available at: www.who.int/countries/eth/eth/en/. [Accessed 27 September 2009].
15. Federal Democratic Republic of Ethiopia, Ministry of Health. *Health Sector Development Programme (HSDP III) 2005–2010*. Addis Ababa, 2005. Available at: moh.gov.et/index.php?option=com_remository-&Itemid=47&func=startdown&id=192.
16. World Health Organization. *Scaling Up, Saving Lives*. 2008. Available at: www.who.int/workforcealliance/documents/Global_Health%20FINAL%20REPORT.pdf.
17. Flawed but fair: Brazil health systems reaches out to the poor. *Bull World Health Organ* 2008; **86**. Available at: www.who.int/bulletin/volumes/86/4/08-030408/en/index.html.
18. Corespondence from Profssor Gilbert [in press].
19. African Union. *Progress Report on the AU Decade for Traditional Medicine (2001–2010). Meeting of experts 4–6 May 2009*. Report number: CAMH/EXP/4(IV). Available at: www.africa-union.org/root/UA/Conferences/2009/mai/SA/04-08mai/CAMH-EXP-4(IV)%20Traditional%20Medicine.doc.

20. Lehmann U, Sanders D. *Community health workers: What do we know about them?* World Health Organization, 2006. Available at: www.hrhresourcecenter.org/node/1587.
21. Haines A, Sanders D, Lehmman U et al. Achieving child survival goals: potential contribution of community health workers. *The Lancet* 2007; **369**: 2121–31.
22. Bang AT, Bang RA, Baitule SB, Reddy MH, Deshmukh MD. Effect of home-based neonatal care and management of sepsis on neonatal mortality: field trial in rural India. *Lancet* 1999; **354**: 1955–61.
23. Lady Health Worker Programme. *External Evaluation of the National Programme for the Family Planning and Primary Health Care. Quantitative Survey Report.* Islamabad: Oxford Policy Management, 2002.
24. Zhang D, Unschuld PU. China's barefoot doctor: past, present and future. *The Lancet* 2008; **372**: 1865–1867.
25. Frenk J. Bridging the divide: global lessons from evidence-based health policy in Mexico. *Lancet* 2006; **368**: 954–961.
26. Natchiar G, Thulasiraj RD, Meenakshi Sundaram R. Cataract surgery at Aravind Eye Hospitals: 1988–2008. *Community Eye Health* 2008; **2**: 40–2.
27. Rosen A. Destigmatizing day-to-day practices: What Can Developed Countries learn from Developing Countries? *World Psychiatry* 2006; **5**: 21–24. Available at: www.pubmedcentral.nih.gov/articlerender.fcgi?artid=1472257.
28. Sirkin HL, Hemerling JW, Bhattacharya AK. *Globality – Competing with Everyone from Everywhere for Everything.* New York: Business Plus, 2008.
29. Mawson A. *The Social Entrepreneur – making communities work.* London: Atlantic Pub, 2008.
30. The Directorate for Health and Social Affairs. Ministry of Health and Care Services, Oslo, Norway. *Recruitment of Health Workers: Towards Global Solidarity.* Report number: IS-1490E, 2007. Available at: www.helsedirektoratet.no/vp/multimedia/archive/00018/IS-1490E_18611a.pdf.
31. World Health Organization. *Treat, Train, Retain – Task Shifting: rational redistribution of tasks among health workforce teams; Global recommendations and guidelines.* 2008. Available at: www.who.int/healthsystems/TTR-TaskShifting.pdf.
32. Department of Health. *The NHS Plan: A plan for investment, a plan for reform.* 2001. Available at: www.dh.gov.uk/en/Publications/PublicationsPolicyAnd Guidance/DH_4002960.
33. The Tropical Health & Education Trust. Available at: www.thet.org.
34. MEMISA. Available at: www.memisa.be/Public/SousRubrique.php?ID=82&language=eng.
35. ESTHER. Available at: www.esther.fr.
36. Leatherman S. [Personal communication]. 28 September 2006.

7 Practical knowledge for the twenty-first century (1) – people and patients

Some Muslim communities in India refuse to have their children immunised by, what they see as, the Hindu authorities. They apparently fear that the immunisation programme is really a sterilisation programme in disguise, designed to keep their population down.

This story, which I heard whilst travelling in India, immediately reminded me of a similar occasion when people didn't trust the authorities in my own country. There was a storm of controversy in the UK when a researcher claimed that the measles, mumps and rubella (MMR) immunisation programme was linked to an increased incidence of autism. His claim caused a large number of parents in the UK to decide not to have their children immunised with the MMR.

Other researchers and the medical leadership and authorities as a whole emphatically rejected his research and his findings.

I worked in the Department of Health at the time and know how hard we tried to persuade parents that there was no reason to fear MMR immunisation. Indeed, we argued that their children would be at greater risk if they weren't vaccinated and caught measles. Whilst it may appear to be a normal childhood disease, measles can and does kill. We were worried that immunisation levels would fall amongst the population and that we would see an upsurge in disease.

On this occasion the politicians, civil servants and managers deliberately took a supporting role; whilst the medical and nursing professions, which enjoyed much higher levels of public trust, made the argument in print, television and media and in clinics and surgeries throughout the country.

Sir Liam Donaldson, the Chief Medical Officer, led the campaign. He has a very good presence in the media and was at his most rational and reassuring in his role as the nation's doctor. His 'bed-side' manner was faultless. So too, I have no doubt, was the approach taken by thousands of doctors and nurses who advised parents in their surgeries and clinics.

We failed.

We failed to convince sufficient numbers of parents that we were right and the researcher was wrong. As a result around 15% of children in London were not vaccinated. Measles is back in the city. Measles is killing again.

This wasn't an argument about science. We had all the scientific knowledge we needed. We just didn't know how to make people believe us. Ultimately, as in India, it was about trust.

History in India may have taught the Muslim villagers not to trust the authorities. History too, sadly, has taught similar lessons in the UK and in other rich countries. We were trapped in an 'us' and 'them' situation. We knew the science; they knew that the authorities weren't always to be trusted.

Myths and realities

Both this and the next chapter are about the practical knowledge that is needed to improve health in the twenty-first century. They build on the knowledge and insights of the twentieth century but show how they need to be adapted in practice to meet the new challenges. This chapter is about people, patients and society, whilst the next deals with scientific knowledge and systems. Both draw on experience and evidence from around the world, from richer and poorer countries alike.

The first part of this chapter looks at how health professionals and planners, for all their scientific and professional knowledge, may not be able to get patients to do what they need to do to improve their own health. It exposes some of the myths about the relationships between patients and professionals. It discusses trust, looks at how patients make their own decisions about health, at how culture determines their behaviour and how social and health issues are inevitably intertwined. It shows that patients are in reality very far from being the patient patients that western scientific medicine assumes that they are.

The second part looks at some of the approaches that have been taken to capitalise on and cope with this independence of mind: from educating the public to 'nudging' them in the right direction and from creating 'expert patients' to 'empowering' patients to improve their own health.

The chapter concludes by returning to some of the lessons learned from poorer countries about social enterprises and self-help and links them with some of the experiences of people in richer countries. It argues that ultimately people want independence to live their own lives and that good health is an important part of this.

The white coats strategy

I think that many clinicians were genuinely shocked and bewildered by the fact that they couldn't persuade every parent to allow their children to have the MMR vaccine. They saw themselves as different. Politicians and managers might not be trusted, but as doctors and nurses they expected to have the confidence of their patients and the public.

These stories illustrate how the environment in which professionals practice and policymakers plan is changing profoundly. We can't just go on doing what we did before and expecting it to work as it did. We tested that out very thoroughly in the case of MMR. Whilst the controversy raged we tried to find ways of getting even more clinicians and even more health organisations to make public announcements supporting MMR vaccination. We did more of what we were already doing.

We made full use of the 'white coats strategy' of getting clinicians onto the television, preferably dressed for the part in white coats or nurses' uniforms, to try to persuade parents. We turned up the volume. In the end it may have been counterproductive with people wondering why we were so insistent and why it looked like we were trying so hard to silence one voice that dissented from the mainstream.

These stories also illustrate something that is coming much more to the fore in the twenty-first century. At an earlier time people in India might well have been forcibly sterilised. In the UK, parents might not have had so much influence over what happened to them and their children. British children might just have been vaccinated, perhaps at school, as part of a national programme without parents being asked for their permission.

Now, however, we all have different expectations of our relationship with authority and with authority figures in every area of life. We are living in a world where our demands for greater openness and democracy have been strengthened by the ease of communication, the availability of information and increasing global emphasis on human rights. Policy makers and academics, such as Sir Leszek Borysiewicz of the Medical Research Council and Dr Heidi Larson of Imperial College, London, are now developing ideas and proposals for new approaches to implementation and improving trust.[1,2]

The MMR story was further complicated because the Prime Minister, Tony Blair, refused to say whether his young son had had the vaccine. As a parent it was perfectly appropriate that he would want to protect his family's privacy. Once questions of this sort are asked, questioners will undoubtedly want to come back more and more often for more and more intrusive information. However, it didn't help the Government's argument.

In a different age, of course, people would not have dreamed of questioning a Prime Minister in this way and they would have listened more trustingly to their doctors.

People talk variously about 'the death of deference' or a 'fracturing of traditional society'. Whatever the causes, the reality is that we increasingly expect to hold those in authority, whoever they are, to account. We want to question and decide for ourselves. We won't just take their knowledge on trust. They won't take ours.

Moreover, we are more likely to take our opinions and our beliefs from our peers, from those people we see as 'just like us'.

Patients have the control

The indigenous people of Alaska, the Alaska Natives, have some important things to teach us. I became exposed to their thinking through Doug Eby, the South Central Foundation (SCF) senior physician executive, who works for them. He and others from SCF speak about their transformed system of care that now provides very good outcomes for significantly less cost. They believe that clinicians and people running heath services don't pay anything like enough attention to what patients think and, even more importantly, what they do. Their system is customer-owned, customer-designed, customer-driven - at both the individual and system level.

In most medical systems the authorities, the clinicians and the managers, don't think about how patients are going to apply their own beliefs and their knowledge, however accurate or inaccurate they may be.

Doug is a doctor who went to Alaska more than a decade ago to work in support of the Alaska Native run health system and has settled into a community made up of Alaska Native people, non-Native individuals, adventurers and oilmen. He maintains that, based on long conversations with the SCF patient community, that whatever their doctor says, in most cases the patient is going to decide what will happen next. All his experience, in Alaska and other parts of the United States, tells him this.

He and SCF point out that it is only in relatively extreme high acuity cases that the professional is fully in charge of the situation and can get the patient to do everything he or she wants. This is true Doug explains, when the patient is in a coma, anesthetised or collapsed; but the lesser the symptoms, the greater the chance that the patient will do what he or she wants to do and will take the professional's advice selectively at best.

Doug argues forcefully that we have to understand this relationship between the acuity of the patient's condition and the amount of autonomy they exercise. I still have the line drawing he sketched to show me just how simple the relationship is. He subsequently sent

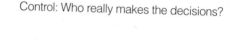

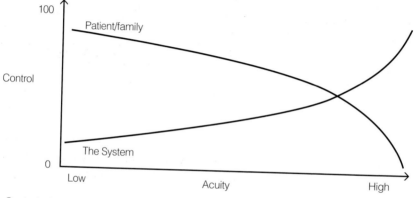

1. Control who makes the final decision influencing outcomes?
2. Influences family, friends, co-workers, religion, values, money
3. Real opportunity to influence health costs/outcomes influence on the choices made behavorial change
4. Current model tests, diagnosis, treatment (medication or procedures)

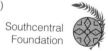

Southcentral
Foundation

Figure 7.1 South Central Foundation, Alaska

me the more refined SCF drawing shown in Figure 7.1, which shows there is a crossover point from patient to clinician control.

"Health professionals simply won't be able to do our jobs properly", Doug says very firmly, "if we succumb to the myth that people normally obey doctor's orders". They don't. As patients, we don't.

Many health care planners and clinicians talk about the importance of empowering patients. They generally mean by this giving people the knowledge and the skills to look after themselves, have choices and make decisions. They mean that clinicians shouldn't just do things to and for patients. These are all very important points but SCF's drawing shows that we are starting in the wrong place. We need to see the world the other way up and start by recognising that in general patients have the control.

Looking at this the other way up we can see that, too often, the behaviours of clinicians and the way systems work tend to disempower patients. This happens in all sorts of both subtle and obvious ways.

The language used by clinicians and the environment of hospitals and clinics may be alien and intimidating. As patients, we may feel disempowered because we are dealing with people who know so much more than we do and with institutions that seem to embody all the knowledge of science. The chances are that when we go to see a professional we are probably already anxious about our health. With our confidence dented by our surroundings, we may not have the courage to mention those other symptoms, which may be minor or they may not be, or to ask the questions that are really worrying us. There may not even be time to do so.

Most clinicians understand these points very well and medical and nursing schools have reflected them in their education for 20 years and longer. However, in practice our health systems don't reflect them and patients often don't experience them in reality.

We may be lucky enough to get a clinician who listens to our story and reflects on our insights into the problem. We may easily not. Even if we do, however, we may both find it difficult to communicate with each other and we may find that the system makes it harder for the clinician to respond.

Dr Beverley, whose work in New York was described in Chapter 6, puts it very well. Clinicians have to work very hard indeed to communicate and understand what the patient is not saying as well as what they are.

There are really three practical questions here for clinicians and for health planners: how to empower patients, how not to disempower them and the deeper question of how to secure their trust sufficiently for them to empower the professionals?

The people of Jimma

Patients very often refuse, in practice, to take on the role that the health system ascribes to them of being the passive as well as patient recipients of services. People make their own trade-offs and decide what they are going to do based on what is important to them.

There are many reasons, of course, why what patients think and know may be very different from what clinicians think and know and why they may act very differently from how clinicians and planners may like them to. It is not just about lack of trust or about different knowledge. It is about a whole range of perceptions and beliefs. These may mean that patients don't even look for help in the first place or accept it when it is offered.

This doesn't just happen in richer western countries, where social changes linked to greater affluence and better education are producing generations of people accustomed to questioning authority. It has probably always happened, although perhaps in a less visible way, as the following example from Ethiopia suggests.

A research project in Ethiopia looked in some detail at this question of why patients didn't seek care when they needed it. The researchers worked in and around Jimma, the town where I met Dr Beed, the Consultant Intensivist from Nottingham, as I described in Chapter 1. Jimma is an agricultural and university centre with a population of around

160 000 in the southwest of the country. The inhabitants are generally poor, although the warmer wetter climate of this area means that the land is more fertile and the population aren't as poor as in the highlands of the north.

There is a university hospital in the town and, whilst Ethiopia has only about US$5 per head per annum to fund its services, there is a range of services available. In these circumstances the researchers wondered why so many people, particularly from the countryside, failed to seek help for conditions that could be dealt with by the local health system.[3]

The researchers asked about three things:

1. the patients' perception of illness: what did they think about the severity of the illness and did they have any idea of the long-term implications and the support they might need?

2. the quality of the health service: did patients believe the treatment was worthwhile and would work?; Did they think it was easy to get treated and how did the staff treat them?

3. the costs of seeking treatment: did they have to pay for treatment; were there travel costs to meet and would they lose income by taking time off work?

The researchers concluded that patients were much more likely to seek care when they understood the severity of the illness, appreciated the quality of the service and believed that the benefits of treatment outweighed the costs. Whether or not they sought help depended on their perceptions, beliefs and knowledge.

These findings, shown in Figure 7.2, might well apply equally in the UK or the USA. There are many accounts of patients not seeking care when they need it, put off by cost or long queues, or by not realising how serious their problem was. I have come across many instances where people don't seek help or where they don't value the help they are given. The result is often that resources are wasted with patients not attending clinic appointments or not taking the medications they have been given.

Patients make their decisions on their perceptions of:

- *Severity of the illness*
- *Quality of the service*
- *Whether the benefits outweigh the costs*

Figure 7.2 Patients' judgements and trade-offs in considering seeking care

Studies suggest that between 30% and 50% of patients don't take their prescription medicine in full and that the annual cost of wasted drugs in the UK is about £100 million.[4] The Medical Director of one Blue Cross organisation, a health insurance business, in the USA told me that their research showed that as many as 30% of people didn't even fill the prescriptions they had been given. They simply didn't take the prescription to the pharmacy and purchase the drugs.

Part of this was because of the cost, but another big part, he thought, was that the patients simply hadn't been convinced that the drugs were worthwhile or worth the trade-offs between their cost and effort and the likely benefit. They made their own decision on the facts as they saw them. Researchers in the UK make a similar analysis, although costs do not play such a significant role.[5]

The way that people behave isn't by any means straightforward or necessarily consistent. Some people may ignore the doctor's advice to change their lifestyle. Others may not take their prescriptions for any one of a number of reasons from thinking they don't need them to reasoning that they probably don't work to not understanding what they are meant to do to forgetting about them or simply being too lazy.

Others, of course, may go out of their way to seek and follow advice, self-prescribe, buy health foods and supplements and adhere to the strictest of healthy regimes. Commerce and the media help them to do this by constantly reminding them of their anxieties and marketing to them the newest products and ideas. The formal health system of doctors, hospitals and prescription drugs is a multibillion dollar industry but so too is the informal health economy of healthy living, diets, supplements, exercise and meditation.

The point here is very simple: every patient is different and everyone is an individual whose behaviour and beliefs affect the way health professionals can care for them. Patients, consciously or unconsciously, make the big decisions.

The primary diagnosis is social

In this chapter we have started to confront the fact that if health professionals are to apply their knowledge successfully they need to be capable of dealing with all the uncertainties of trust, belief and perception as well as recognising, respecting and working with the fact that every patient has his or her own autonomy and, unless professionals disempower them, makes their own decisions. This takes us into a world where professionals in rich countries may need to think more like people in poor ones.

The Alaska Native SCF experience and thinking can once again offer us insight. They listen and learn from the community they serve, in fact they talk a lot about being customer-driven and customer-designed. They also draw on generations of wisdom held by the tribal elders about what makes people do what they do and how to influence them to do it differently.

Tall and very forceful, SCF's Doug Eby is a compelling speaker. I have seen him address audiences; lecture may be a better word for the energy, passion and certainty he puts into his views and the views of the Alaska native community about the need to concentrate on a patient's social circumstances. He has learned from native leaders and as a clinician, he tells us, that for many patients "The primary diagnosis is social".

His, SCF's point, is crushingly simple. The old man may have Parkinson's but his biggest and most immediate problem is that he is isolated, lonely, not eating and washing properly and starting to wander physically and mentally. You should deal, SCF believes, with the personal and family social issues as the primary diagnosis and, then only as part of the whole package, treat the Parkinson's. Most patients, the worried well and the genuinely sick alike, they assert are like this.

I have been in audiences of clinicians and health managers who have loved every word Doug and his colleagues have spoken and enjoyed his style and presentation, but I have wondered if after all the stimulation and entertainment they went back to running their own old systems in their old ways.

It must seem very difficult to work out how you are going to employ this insight back home in the well-structured environment of a healthcare system geared to treating the illness. Everyone working in healthcare is familiar with the difficult problems that people with significant social problems create: the homeless, the addicts, the misfits, the elderly people who have deteriorated to the point where they can't go home and have no carers to look after them.

SCF has applied their thinking in their own area and have produced their own much more sophisticated version of the simple 'lifebelt' model I described in Chapter 3, where the patient at the centre can draw on services from different areas as they are needed. It can be done and Doug and colleagues are doing it. The Alaska Native SCF model believes that we should start thinking about all our patients, not just this group, as if the first concern, the primary diagnosis, was their social situation. If we do so, we will change the way we design their services.

There are many reasons why people don't apply the SCF approach in practice. After all, they may even want to rationalise, they are working in a very different location. Other people don't behave like the Alaska Native people. Social issues aren't as important.

Few healthcare systems in rich countries, if any, are geared to taking social factors fully into account. Their concern is for the acutely ill not the chronically ill. Health systems are resourced to look after people when they are in the acute phases of illness. They are not generally able or willing to deal with the longer term problems of rehabilitation or, for example, to help an elderly lady weakened by her illness live safely at home.

"We are not social workers" I have heard some hospital doctors complain when faced with a patient of this sort. "This isn't our business."

It is, however, fast becoming our business.

As we saw earlier in Chapter 3 about *Health and wealth,* the so-called 'lifestyle diseases', associated with our behaviour and our appetites, are increasing and clinicians treating us will need to understand more about our social situation. The increase in chronic diseases and the ageing of the population in rich countries will make us need to focus on how to provide continuing support for middle-aged and elderly people as they have periods of acute illness and come in and out of hospital over the years.

SCF is right. We need to pay much more attention to the social diagnosis.

This has become our business.

Society and culture

The story of the research in Jimma was also about culture. It was about how people thought about their illness. Did they see it simply as a physical phenomenon or did they perhaps think that someone or something caused it? Was it retribution or punishment? What about the treatment that was on offer? Did people believe in the medicines available?

Culture, beliefs, traditions and ways of looking at the world all affect what we believe we know and how we act. These questions aren't new. Benjamin David Paul, for many the founding father of medical anthropology in the USA, wrote in 1955:

"If you wish to help a community improve its health, you must learn to think like the people of the community. Before asking a group of people to assume new health habits, it is wise to ascertain the existing habits, how these habits are linked to one another, what functions they perform, and what they mean to those who practice them."[6]

All the aspects of habits that Paul draws attention to are important. Our beliefs and habits don't exist in isolation from everything else about us. Improving health is not as simple as just changing one belief or one habit.

Susan Scrimshaw, now President of the Sage Colleges in the USA, illustrates this in writing about efforts to treat HIV/AIDS in Sub-Saharan Africa. She draws attention to gender roles and different cultural traditions, describing how it is the different combinations of cultural, social and economic factors that can make it so difficult to treat AIDS patients and restrict its spread.[7]

She describes the secrecy regarding HIV/AIDS that is common within the region. It is a source of shame and something to be denied, as it is indeed in most cultures of the world. She also draws attention to specific examples of how people think about AIDS. In some areas, for example, there is a superstition that having sex with a virgin will cure an HIV-infected man. In other areas it is seen as a curse from the gods resulting from the people having adopted western ways.

These perceptions can manifest themselves in many different ways. In parts of southern Africa, for example, women don't register for antenatal care because they know that they will be tested for HIV/AIDS and that, if they prove positive, they will be ostracised and perhaps abandoned by their husband, family and friends. The stigma is so powerful that they risk their lives and health not only from increased risk in childbirth but also, if they are HIV positive, by forgoing the treatment.

The difficulty in tackling AIDS in South Africa was made worse for many years because the Health Minister and President denied the existence of AIDS as a separate condition and argued it could be dealt with by diet and other non-medical approaches. The truth is that cultural and behavioural approaches are needed alongside medical treatment and drugs. The South African Government set back AIDS treatment in their country by many years.

Culture is not always a barrier. It can also accelerate health.

Dr Janet Smylie works as a doctor with people from the First Nations, Métis and Inuit communities in Canada and is developing ways to make sure that their knowledge and beliefs can be used alongside western scientific medicine to improve health and contribute to the wider goal of 'indigenous success.'

I was privileged to hear her talk about her work at a conference in Vancouver that the British Columbian Government was hosting as part of a process for creating a new vision and new plans for health in the Province. Young and passionate, she is Métis herself and able to speak with the authority of being both insider and outsider. She has access to local knowledge and to the whole output of western scientific medicine to help her in her quest.[8]

Her aim in the talk was to raise awareness of the needs of indigenous communities and encourage the BC Government to work alongside them to ensure that health services fitted with local health knowledge and systems. Whilst her aim was local, her messages were global. Put simply, there were three of them.

Firstly, health needs to be seen as part of the wider picture and wider goals. It doesn't stand alone. She saw it as contributing to indigenous success or, in the words of Professor Mason Durie, a public health expert from New Zealand, helping create indigenous resilience and moving from disease and disadvantage to the realisation of potential.[9] Improving health was about improving life more generally.

Secondly, this could only happen if everything done to improve health was fully aligned with all other aspects of their society such as family relationships and cultural and religious beliefs. Working to tackle a particular disease, for example, wouldn't work well and might even be counterproductive unless all the actions fitted in with other things that were happening. Communities could well reject the efforts, as we saw in the earlier examples from India and Ethiopia, for any one of many different reasons of trust, beliefs or perceptions.

Thirdly, and specifically, health professionals needed to consider all the different sorts of evidence they were presented with, the social as well as the scientific, and to find ways to evaluate how they can be used to improve health.

These three messages may seem to be very much common sense and as if they should apply to every health system in rich or poor countries. In reality they are not how most health systems operate. Individual clinicians may well try to take account of all of these factors; however, the health systems within which they work in rich countries will, typically, focus on the disease or condition and pay little or no attention to the rest of a patient's life.

The community vision held by the people of Kahnawake and quoted by Dr Smylie draws together all the aspects of a healthy life from diet and exercise to the relationships with family and the environment:

"All Kahnawakero:non are in excellent health. Diabetes no longer exists. All the children and adults eat healthily at all meals and are physically active daily. The children are actively supported by their parents and family who provide nutritious food obtainable from family gardens, local food distributors and the natural environment. The schools as well as community organisations, maintain programs and policy that reflect and reinforce healthy eating habits and daily physical activity. There are a variety of physical activities for all people offered at a range of recreational facilities in the community. All people accept the responsibility to cooperatively maintain a well community for the future Seven Generations."

Education, engagement and empowerment

Not all communities take their health as seriously as the Kahnawakero:non appear to do and many individuals, including many of those most at risk, ignore their health and live unhealthy lifestyles. Health policymakers who have a responsibility to improve health need to find the best ways to, on the one hand respect and work with people's autonomy and, on the other, encourage, nudge and empower the public towards healthy behaviour.

This chapter can only offer a very brief survey of some of the many creative ways in which people have worked to educate, engage and empower people. There are many ap-

Policymakers have worked through:

- *Education and social marketing*
- *Supporting expert parents and expert patients*
- *Engaging patients directly in their own care*
- *Consulting and listening*
- *Responding to politics and social action*

Figure 7.3 Engaging the public in health improvement

proaches as outlined in Figure 7.3. Here we will look here at some of those that involve trying to change people's behaviour. Ultimately, however, as I shall argue, they will not be fully successful unless they genuinely transfer power to the public and patients – to go with the ultimate decision-making power that they already have.

We start with health education and marketing. In many countries there is a long tradition of health promotion campaigns through which governments, public bodies and charities seek to influence public behaviour, with varying degrees of success. They work alongside health educators in schools and parenting and other programmes run by health organisations.

Internationally, non-smoking campaigns have used a mixture of campaigning with the public to change their behaviour and legislation to restrict advertising and smoking in public places. This has, after many years, brought about significant changes of behaviour amongst some populations in richer countries, but not all. In much of Sub-Saharan Africa the focus is on AIDS and sexual practices. Billboards in Uganda proclaim: "Say no to sugar daddies. Stamp out inter-generational sex" as well as, to western eyes, more familiar messages about using condoms. In richer countries they are currently more likely to be about obesity with advice on diet and exercise.

These approaches risk alienating the public with accusations of 'nannying' and patronising people and interfering with people's rights to behave as they wish within the law. The MMR campaign with which we started this chapter is in a long tradition where people in authority have told the public what is good for them. As we saw, it no longer works reliably.

In recent years there has been a development in understanding and knowledge about so-called social marketing through which marketing messages are aligned with social habits and ways of thinking. Particular groups in the population are targeted with specific messages designed just for them. It is much easier to get people to accept a message if it fits in with their preconceptions, habits and beliefs. This approach relies to some extent on the idea that we tend to do and think what our friends do and think and are more inclined to believe, as noted earlier, what we are told by "people like us".

It uses some of the skills of anthropology but also borrows from the experience of commercial organisations such as supermarkets that have identified that peoples' shopping habits tend to conform to regular patterns. People who buy this particular newspaper, for example, may well consume these pre-prepared meals and these alcoholic drinks and take these sorts of holidays. Knowing these patterns allows organisations to target their marketing efforts to best effect on the people who are most likely to want the particular product being marketed.

The NHS has used this approach in marketing health messages. Slough is a large town west of London with a relatively high population of people with a family background in South Asia and who are therefore more susceptible to diabetes than average for the UK. Health planners believed that there were many undiagnosed diabetics in the community who, if they could be diagnosed early enough, would be more treatable and less disabled by the disease. They would also cost the NHS less if their disease was caught early.

The local NHS organisation employed an experienced firm of analysts, normally employed by the big supermarkets, to create a marketing campaign that would use knowledge of peoples' shopping, work and leisure habits to advertise to them in the right way in the right places. This was a very precisely targeted health education campaign designed to reach the groups thought to be most at risk. It was very successful, with many more people identified with diabetes and entering early treatment and management.

These developments in social marketing are becoming more sophisticated all the time with, as I write, the latest theory being that it is more effective to 'nudge' people in the direction you want them to go rather than lecturing them or marketing to them directly. *Nudge: Improving Decisions about Health, Wealth and Happiness* by Richard Thaler and Cass Sunstein, the book that has popularised this idea, takes as one of its examples the problem of how to get people to sign up to their willingness to be organ donors.

Most countries use an opt-in system that requires people to make an explicit decision and carry an organ donor card; some countries have considered making it an opt-out matter, in which it will be assumed that you are willing to be a donor unless you have explicitly said that you aren't. Both systems require a great deal of marketing and effort to get people to make a decision. *Nudge* suggests a better idea: put the question on the form that people have to complete to tax their car each year. This way there is no extra effort involved, people can very easily respond.[10]

This raises the question of how can we make healthy living the easy option?

The expert parent and the expert patient

Another approach is to work with people who have themselves become expert over the years on their own diseases, and with mothers – the people who are most likely to be able to affect the health of others and, of course, who are experts on their own children.

Mr Abed's dictum "Empower the women", described in the last chapter, holds good throughout the world. We know that a baby born to a Bolivian mother with no education has a 10% chance of dying, while one born to a woman with at least secondary education has a 0.4% chance. This is a 25-fold difference. A child born in India to a mother with 5 years' education has a 40% better chance of living to 5 years old than a child whose mother has no education.[11]

The crucial fact in these two cases is that the mother has some education: any education, not specifically about health. Even just 5 years' primary education gives the mother a greater ability to think for herself and understand more about the world. It makes the world a safer place for her baby.

Children in rich and poor countries alike receive a wide variety of health education in their schools. As importantly, they can become literate and numerate, learn about science and, most importantly, how to think systematically and logically. The crucial point is that these lessons are designed to help people to think for themselves and make their own judgements about risks and rewards as independent human beings.

American health insurers use financial rewards to help educate their customers and change their behaviour. They have developed incentives over recent years to encourage their customers to keep themselves healthy and have specifically targeted the American 'Mom' with her power to influence what her family does. I recall Jack Lord of Humana and Leonard Schaeffer of Wellpoint, two of the leading health insurance companies in the USA, explaining to a business audience that our mothers were the people who taught us to wash our hands and clean our teeth and that health businesses should make much greater efforts to reach them. Mothers are the great educators. For Humana and Well-point this was good health and just plain good business sense. For mothers in Africa using their knowledge about clean water and insecticide-treated mosquito bed nets is a matter of life and death.

It is not surprising that clinicians, policymakers and businessmen who wish to improve health want to understand how to influence parents and patients alike. There are schemes and projects and policies in every part of the world designed variously to educate and to empower. Surestart in the UK, based partly on ideas developed in the USA, is designed to help mothers give their children the best start in life with health as a key component.

Other programmes make use of the patient's own expertise. In the UK, for example, the Expert Patient programme worked with patients with chronic diseases, such as arthritis or chronic obstructive pulmonary disease, and who understand their own condition very well to help others to learn about how to control their condition and to train professional staff. In Uganda, in a scheme with some similarities, women with AIDS are employed to work with AIDS patients. They bring to their work an understanding that is different but complementary to the professionals.

These sorts of approaches are even more important where there are minority groups within a dominant majority culture. Health workers who are culturally attuned to the group they are working with can reach more of the population and understand how best to link the needs of this group into the wider health system, which will no doubt reflect the culture and practices of the majority. Asian women are more likely to be able to influence other Asian women about diet and exercise. Patients from the same group, people like us, may be the most effective health tutors after, of course, our mothers.

People, however expert, aren't always able to get their messages across or to influence policy and help shape services. Polly Arango lives in New Mexico, where she and her husband look after their son, Nick, who is 33 years old and has a progressive neurological condition without a name. Nick cannot walk or talk, and, in Polly's words, "has a seizure disorder, is fed by a g-tube, must be suctioned often at night, and requires care 24/7. He weighs less than 70 pounds and is considered medically fragile."

Over the years Polly has become a true expert on her son's condition and on what sort of services people like him need. She faced difficulties at every turn but ultimately was able to put together a package of the support Nick needed. As a result of her own experiences she became the Co-founder and, for a long period, Executive Director of Family Voices, a network of more than 45 000 families and friends whose aim is to improve health and related systems for children and youths with special health needs. She is now listened to in national fora and her advice is sought by any number of policymakers and health leaders. There are other people around the world who could tell other stories of fighting to be heard. Some have had Polly's success. Some haven't.

Now, as I write in autumn 2009, Polly has just told me about Nick's latest problems. He has started to experience new symptoms and has once again been passed around the system from Emergency room to consulting room and back. At every step Polly has told the clinicians about his history and her knowledge of what he needs. At every step she has been ignored. She will get what Nick needs eventually, of course. She won't stop until she has done. In the meantime, even someone as fearless, determined, knowledgeable and expert as Polly has found herself being disempowered.

The messages from all these schemes for policymakers are similar. They are simple and straightforward. They should empower. They should enable people to get an education and think for themselves. They should also stop disempowering people by treating them as passive recipients of their wisdom and treat them as fellow citizens and experts in their own right.

Full engagement

It can be very difficult for patients' groups and individuals to get attention or to influence services. Most countries that have some form of public health system have a formal way to involve local people or their elected representatives in decision making and give a popular or, even, democratic legitimacy to policy and plans. This doesn't mean however that it is easy to influence what happens, as Polly Arango, Family Voices and the thousands of advocacy groups around the world can testify.

The engagement of patients and the public in health and healthcare was central to government policy during much of my time as Chief Executive of the NHS. It was based on the understanding that this could not only improve health but also help manage costs.

In 2001 Derek Wanless, a prominent British banker, was asked by the UK Government to examine future health trends and identify the factors determining the long-term financial and resource needs of the NHS to 2002. He developed three scenarios: 'slow uptake', where new technologies and drugs were only brought into use slowly; 'solid progress', where technology and costs grew together; and the 'fully engaged' scenario, where patients themselves contributed much more to improving their health and healthcare.

Wanless concluded that this 'fully engaged' scenario would not only produce the best health outcomes but would be the least expensive. Patients who adopted healthy lifestyles would be healthier and incur fewer healthcare costs, whilst the evidence showed that patients who were directly involved in their care often had better outcomes and used less medication. The report was adopted by the Government and became part of the justification for a substantial increase in funding for the NHS.[12]

This and other reports contributed to a spate of innovations in the NHS that included the use of patients' panels to help determine policy in contentious areas, the involvement of patients' representatives on policy bodies, changes in practice towards greater shared care between patient and doctor, the offering of more choice to patients over their treatment and the development of more 'expert patient'-type schemes around the country. Some of these approaches were very successful but there were practical difficulties, which, whilst they were particular to the NHS, have wider relevance.

My observation as Chief Executive was that there were three practical difficulties. Firstly, this wasn't our only major policy. We were also committed to a massive improvement in every aspect of the quality of the service we gave: from reducing waiting times to improving clinical outcomes and expanding services. These service issues were of much more immediate interest to the public, and therefore the politicians, much more likely to show fast improvements and much simpler to measure. As a result they were in reality given higher priority, received the most attention and saw the most progress achieved.

The second problem was that, whilst service improvements could have been made with a greater focus on patient involvement – and some were – health systems like ours were very heavily invested in traditional practices, which generally excluded patient involvement. These practices were reinforced by how staff had been trained and how our systems for everything from making referrals to policymaking had been designed.

Underlying these two problems was the point that our business models and the way that money was allocated and spent simply didn't encourage or even allow for greater patient involvement. Like most health systems the NHS has fairly rigid ways of paying for service. Healthcare providers would be paid for certain sorts of services, such as inpatient admissions or consultation with a doctor, but would receive nothing extra for engaging patients, consulting, making extra phone calls or providing advice on self-care. Indeed, if this self-care advice was so successful that the patient no longer needed admission, the hospital would lose the income this would have provided. There was a financial disincentive.

These practical problems meant that making significant change would be a massive cultural, financial and logistical exercise. We put enormous effort into service improvements, changing service design and business models as needed. As a result we saw major service improvements. We didn't make the same efforts with patient engagement and, as a result, the improvements in this area were generally fairly limited in scope and marginal in impact.

We were not as radical here as we were in other areas. We needed to turn the world upside down.

Turning the world upside down

The *Wanless Report* was very significant in making the economic as well as the health case for greater patient engagement. We have not yet followed it through by creating the right business models to implement it properly. The UK has, however, in recent years developed its thinking further by finding ways to give people some control over the money spent directly on their health and by offering greater support to social enterprise schemes. Both have echoes of what is happening in poorer countries.

Some disabled and seriously ill people in the UK now receive 'direct payments', which allow them to buy the services they consider they need to help them. They choose between, for example, spending the money on aids for independent living or on extra care. They can select and employ their own carer directly, rather than simply having the one picked for them by the authorities. They have greater autonomy and independence.

This approach has similarities with developments around the world, where people have been using money to incentivise changes in behaviour and increase patient control. Mexico has been a pioneer in conditional cash transfers, as we saw in the last chapter, giving payments directly to very poor parents to improve the diet and care of their children. Bangladesh now offers money to expectant mothers when they attend antenatal clinics. Singapore, uniquely amongst the nations of the world, has a health system based almost entirely on personal budgets. American insurance companies, as we have seen, offer incentives for personal action to improve health.

The basic concept of giving people money to deal with their immediate needs is not new in any of the countries that have had some form of welfare state. Parents receive child benefits in the UK and the equivalent in other countries to help with costs of child rearing. There are unemployment benefits and disability allowances. All these schemes give the recipient some power to spend the money as they see fit, unlike the type of programmes more familiar in the USA, where vouchers or items of food, clothing and furniture may be provided but recipients have limited discretion over spending.

The difference is that, for really the first time, these ideas are being tried in health where the professions and the institutions have for so long controlled the purse strings and held the power. They directly challenge the status quo.

There are risks with this approach. The schemes in Mexico were only introduced after careful study and the evaluation of pilots. There need, for example, to be safeguards to manage the obvious risk that the money might be used for other purposes.

These approaches may also introduce new risks. We need only look at the way consumers who pay for their own healthcare are so much at the mercy of the commercial producers to understand the need for some regulation and control. The very poorest and worst educated might not be able to exercise this control and would be at further disadvantage. Others, well educated, may not want to take on this level of responsibility, seeing it as adding to their worries and anxieties.

The approach of direct payments can only ever be a part of the solution in health. Another part may be found in something else we are familiar with from poorer countries: social enterprises. The UK has a tradition of social enterprises, as mentioned briefly in the last chapter, where organisations have used business methods to achieve social aims with pioneers working in housing, social welfare, education and health. The most successful have worked in all these fields, recognising that social issues cross across them all. There has been an upsurge recently in interest in these sorts of organisations and the NHS has deliberately set out to help create such bodies.

As yet, and largely for the reasons I gave earlier to explain the relatively poor progress with patient engagement, they have not had much impact. The NHS has other more immediate priorities; the systems and the professionals are not geared towards these ideas and there isn't yet a suitable business model. It is not just that NHS planning, commissioning and payment systems work against them. The problem is also that health, social services and housing expenditure is managed separately.

These sorts of rigidities, both internally within health and externally across sectors, are mirrored in other countries where payment methods as well as training and systems get in the way of seeing a patient's problems in the round.

As we saw from Doug Eby's experience, the primary diagnosis is very often social. Patients, after all, are very often people with many needs. The day-to-day problems for anyone trying to address a patient's housing, social and health needs all at the same time are immense and give health and social workers enormous difficulties throughout the world. BRAC addresses this sort of issue in Bangladesh with health groups, training programmes to help women set up their small enterprises, a BRAC bank to help finance them and outlets to help sell produce. They try to help people to stand on their own feet and manage their own futures.

These approaches – of direct payments and the development of social enterprises – are in their infancy in the UK. Nevertheless they break with the paternal traditions of the professions and government and seem to be able to contribute to so many of the things we have discussed in this chapter. They acknowledge patient control, knowledge and expertise. They avoid the immediate issues of trust and accountability. They respect the patient's right to make decisions within their own cultural context. They seem to be particularly suited to patients with long-term and chronic conditions, whom, as we know, are the major users of the health service.

One of the major steps to take now must be to develop the business model that reflects better the reality of patient control. When that happens we will begin to see that we have moved from professionals wishing to empower patients and to stop disempowering them to a situation where professionals are empowered to work on their behalf by patients and communities.

We need new business models if we are to turn the world upside down, but we also need to understand what it will look like when we have done so. The final example of a patient's experience that I will use in this chapter underlines the point that the patient is best placed to make their own judgements about their own life and health and introduces ideas about human rights.

We are all disabled now

There is a great deal that disabled people can teach us about the right to health and rights in general from their experience and perspective.

Disabled people and disability are a key theme in this book both because many thousands of people are disabled every year in poor countries where accidents and physical trauma take a terrible toll and because there are so many examples of people rising above their disability to inspire others.

There is, however, a perennial danger that policymakers may treat disability as a simple one-dimensional problem in which people need to overcome their particular inability to walk or to see or to hear. It is, of course much more complicated than this. Blindness or mental health can be devastating, throwing a whole family into poverty.

Amartya Sen, the Nobel laureate, argues that policymakers fail to understand the complications and implications of disability because of the way they look at the world; starting, as most of us probably do, with the idea that their policy should be constructed around the needs of 'normal' people with exceptions made for those with disabilities of any kind. The result is that their every policy reinforces the disadvantage experienced by disabled people.[13]

Baroness Jane Campbell of Surbiton is a friend who has influenced my thinking and had a powerful impact on several aspects of UK social policy. She has, amongst other things, helped shape the policy of Direct Payments to disabled people in the UK.

When I was Chief Executive of the NHS I arranged to film an interview with her about her experience of health care and hospitals. I played it to a conference of the Chairs and Chief Executives of all England's hospitals and health authorities as a reminder of how far we were from really being patient centred in our care.

Baroness Campbell has been severely disabled from birth. She is small, with limited movement, regularly needs help with breathing and is all too often admitted to hospital for long periods. She is also very bright with a powerful mind, iron determination and a sense of humour: these being the qualities that make her such a successful social commentator and campaigner and so effective a member of the UK's House of Lords.

She told the camera that on her last stay in hospital she had been in intensive care for a long period. One day as she lay there she heard a doctor say to a nurse that if she 'crashed' there was really no need to resuscitate her as she had such a poor quality of life. Jane was appalled. She would be the judge of her own quality of life.

She acted. She made herself stay awake for the next 48 hours so that she could keep an eye on the staff and sent her husband home to get a picture of her receiving her PhD to place at the end of the bed. The person in the picture was whom the doctor was talking about, she said; he shouldn't be misled by the appearance of the poor person struggling with her illness in the bed before him.

Nine hundred powerful men and women stayed very still and silent when the film had finished. I didn't need to say anything. Baroness Campbell had exposed some of our most basic assumptions and revealed the way power operated in our hospitals.

A long-term campaigner for the rights of disabled people, she has argued consistently for the transformative public services that will overcome the social inequality that disabled people's experience. She does not want to be viewed as a vulnerable person in need of care but rather as an active, valued citizen in charge of her own life. Disabled people have the same rights as everybody else.

In a lecture at Cambridge University in April 2008 she set out a distinctive new approach saying that:

> "*The challenges we now face demand that our slogan 'Nothing about us without us', must speak less of our separateness and difference and more of our interdependence and connection with others. Critically, it must be about seeking to share control and responsibility, not simply taking control. Redressing injustice still requires a politics of recognition, but this*

should no longer be reduced to a question of group identity or allegiance. It requires a politics aimed at overcoming barriers that prevent all individuals, families and communities participating as full members of society".[14]

Her very powerful argument is that:

"*the ideas of the disability movement – barrier removal, reforming public services to give people greater control over their own lives, and equality legislation based on accommodating difference rather than ignoring it – are the blueprint for the next stages of promoting equality and human rights overall*".[14]

Jane Campbell was suggesting that, if we threw away our preconceptions, we could learn from her experience and adopt her perspective as someone who, like her, valued and benefited from equality and rights. We may not all be disabled in the conventional sense of the world, but we all have special needs.

She has, in the theme of this book, turned the world upside down.

Independence as the ultimate goal

This chapter has discussed some of the sorts of practical knowledge needed to improve health in the twenty-first century. It seems reasonable to ask what our ultimate goal is. We may acquire much better knowledge about how to improve health, but what are we really aiming for? If we don't know, how will we know if we are succeeding or failing?

The conventional answer would be couched in terms of health for all, where health is not just the absence of disease but a positive sense of wellbeing in body and mind and, perhaps, spirit and soul as well. The World Health Organization writes of "A state of complete physical and mental and social wellbeing".[15]

Janet Smylie takes the answer further, however, and sees health as not just an end in itself. It is part of indigenous success, a healthy life as part of a successful and resilient way of life. I suspect that Doug Eby, from his experiences in Alaska, would agree. It is an attractive idea.

The answer matters because knowing what we are ultimately aiming for will guide our actions. If we can share the same goal with others, we can unify and align our efforts.

Almost 2500 years ago the Greek philosopher Aristotle wrote about *phronesis*, normally translated as practical wisdom. It was the quality, he said, of understanding both the means and the ends, of understanding both what should be done and how to do it. He distinguished between the clever person who knew how to get things done but not what should be done and the wise person who knew what should be done but not how to do it. Practical wisdom was, he believed, much more valuable than either cleverness or wisdom alone.[16]

These old ideas can immediately conjure up for all of us some very modern images. We can see the clever technocrats of the health systems, on the one hand, devising complex ways for managing problems but seeming to miss the point about what it's all for. We have all seen the results of their work. We can also picture the wise heads on the other hand who know what we should be aiming for, but can infuriate the more practically minded by offering vague and theoretical advice about what needs to be done. We have all seen them, occupying the high and dry moral ground whilst other people wrestle with the practical problems in the messy reality of life.

We need to be careful about how we define our goal. It needs to be sufficiently precise and practical for us to be able to apply our cleverness and measure progress but it must also be sufficiently broad to allow us to adapt it to our own circumstances and beliefs.

Dr Jeremy Cobb, the very independent-minded former Public Health Director for East Berkshire in the UK, believes that the crucial endpoint that health professionals should be working towards is to help people function as independently as possible, physically, psychologically and socially. In the absence of such a unifying end goal, people go their separate ways. I recall him trying in the 1990s to get all the professions to assess their patients in terms of their independence. They mostly didn't like it. The nurses wanted their own assessment and had goals to do with care and comfort. The doctors thought in terms of clinical outcomes; social work, as they saw it, still wasn't their business. Only the occupational therapists really reflected on how their patients would eventually manage to resume their old lives.

I have heard Jeremy rail against the separate professions, the doctors, nurses and therapists who all insisted on assessing patients their own way and, in those days, holding separate notes. It led him into plenty of conflict with his more traditionally minded colleagues. That didn't faze Jeremy. He liked the fight. Years later he believes there has been some progress, but that clinicians and health systems still generally think and talk just in terms of clinical outcomes and the outcomes of care and not in terms of how well the patient can function.

Independence is, in practice, what most of us want for our families and ourselves. We want to be able to live as normally as possible with our diseases and disabilities. We don't want to be 'in care' or dependent on others and we don't want to be forced to be 'carers' earlier than we need be. Jane Campbell's experience reminds us that however disabled we may seem to be to others, we may still want to live and make our own judgements and decisions. We can value life at every stage of it and we can ask our physicians and carers to help us to be as able and as independent as possible at every stage.

We can measure independence and understand it and, crucially, we can apply our own values to it. We alone can judge how much we want to be dependent on relatives and friends and institutions. What may be too much dependence for one person may be independence for another.

In some ways Jeremy Cobb's insistence on the end goal being independence is another version of Doug Ebby's assertion that the primary diagnosis is almost always social. Both men are looking at the individual in the round. Both men are asking: what does that individual really want?

It also resonates with Amartya Sen's view that the goal of international development is for people to have the freedom to live a life that they have reason to value. He does not attempt to judge for them what that life might be or how to judge its value. The important unifying goal is freedom.[13]

We can adapt the same phrasing here and say that in health the goal for people is independence and the freedom to live a life they have reason to value.

Conclusions

This chapter has explored some of the most profound issues to do with our health, our beliefs and our values. It has suggested that professionals and policymakers alike need to have real practical knowledge about how to deal with lack of trust, how best to understand the social and cultural context of their patients, and how to respect and work with patient autonomy and engagement. Many questions remain unanswered but a few things stand out clearly.

Patients are at the centre, not because health professionals have placed them there or empowered them to be there and not because a politician or a policymaker had adopted this as a smart slogan. It is because in reality their decisions, actions and beliefs determine what happens most but not all of the time.

There are exceptions, of course, when a patient is in a coma, very ill or confused. Moreover with some patients and some conditions the professional will always be fully in control. However, most patients and most conditions don't fit this pattern. They are more complex. They have special needs.

Once we accept this idea we can see that there are some profound implications. Patient engagement can no longer be treated as if it were an add-on. Systems will have to be changed and business models created that recognise the patient's own role. Health issues can no longer be treated in isolation from everything else in a person's life. Education, employment, housing and health are intimately linked, so is family and culture.

It is no longer possible, if it ever were, for health professionals to treat patients as passive and as patiently waiting for their expert opinion. They need to take into account a myriad of social and cultural issues and recognise and respect an individual's autonomy and wishes if they are to be successful. In truth this is probably how most professionals think and try to operate in practice, even though the systems they work in so often get in the way.

Finally, the goal of independence unifies so much of what we have discussed in this chapter and will inform our thinking in the remaining ones. In the next chapter we will look at how science and systems can help us deliver better health and greater independence. We will come back in the final chapters to the questions of rights, politics and interdependence and to how we can generate the power and momentum needed to make change in the world.

References

1. Borysiewicz L. *Prevention is better than cure*. Harveian Oration 2009. Royal College of Physicians. London 2009.
2. Cooper LZ, Larson HJ, Katz SL. *Protecting Public Trust in Immunisation*. Pediatrics. 122. 1 July 2008; 1–5.
3. Petricca K, Mamo Y, Haileamlak A, Seid E, Parry E. Barriers to effective follow up treatment of rheumatic heart disease in rural Ethiopia. A grounded theory analysis of the patient experience. [Unpublished paper].
4. Department of Health. *Pharmacy in England: building on strengths – delivering the future*. London: Department of Health, 2008.
5. Crome P, Kelly S, Steel J. Have you taken your tablets this week? *Clinical Medicine* 2009; **9**: February.
6. Paul BD. *Health, Culture and Community*. New York: Russell Sage Foundation, 1955.

7. Scrimshaw, SC. Culture, Behavior & Health, In *International Public Health: Diseases, Programs, Systems and Policies*, M Merson (ed). Gaithersburg, MD: Aspen Publishers. Second Edition: M Merson, R Black, A Mills (eds), Sudbury, MA: Jones and Bartlett Publishers, 2006.
8. Smylie J. BC Conference. Vancouver, Canada, 2007.
9. Durie M. Pacific Region Indigenous Doctors Congress, 2006.
10. Thaler RH,Sunstein CR. *Nudge: Improving decisions about health, wealth and happiness*. New Haven, CT: Yale University Press, 2008.
11. World Health Organization. *Closing the gap in a generation: health equity through action on the social determinants of health*. Commision on Social Determinants of Health. 2008
12. Department of Health. *Securing Our Future Health: taking a long term view – The Wanless Review*, January 2002. Available at: www.dh.gov.uk/en/Publicationsandstatistics/Publications/PublicationsPolicyAnd-Guidance/DH_4009293.
13. Sen A. *Development as Freedom*. New York: Knopf, 1999.
14. Campbell J. Lecture, Cambridge University. 2008
15. World Health Organization. Constitution of the World Health Organization. October 2006. www.who.int/governance/eb/who_constitution_en.pdf.
16. Aristotle. *Nichomachean ethics*. 340–50 BC.

8 Practical knowledge for the twenty-first century (2) – science and systems

I sat in the tiered ranks of a lecture room in the University of Cape Town listening bemused to Professor Eric Topol, the Chief Academic Officer of Scripps Health. He was talking through the very latest science in his speciality of cardiac genetics. I was bemused because, unlike the academics and doctors around me, I was having difficulty keeping up with his flow of words and the accompanying slides.

I had, however, got the message that discoveries were coming quick and fast and that scientists were identifying more and more gene variants that were associated with a particular disease. In due course this might lead to cure or, better still, prevention.

I could have heard something of the same story in many such lecture rooms around the world or read accounts of the extraordinary things that scientists are now able to do. We are almost becoming accustomed to the idea that scientists can now do things we hadn't even thought about and that our grandchildren, if not our children, might live to be 150–200 years old. Science fiction is becoming science fact.

In fact what Professor Topol was describing was still a long way from the daily reality of many of the physicians in the room. They dealt mainly with elderly patients whose treatment was complicated by many different factors from their age and general frailty to their multiple conditions.

Interestingly, however, Professor Topol also suggested some ideas that were very relevant to the reality of their practice. He showed us that mutations in different places on the same gene were sometimes associated with different diseases. In this way some myocardial infarctions are 'related' to diabetes and atrial fibrillation is 'related' to some strokes. These relationships had not been known before and might be very important in how we designed our non-genetic treatments for these conditions. There was some immediate interest for today's clinicians.[1]

Towards the end of the lecture I could see that other members of his audience were becoming bemused and amused as he took us to the very edge of the application of his science, way beyond where scientists are normally comfortable going. We were in new territory, where businesses were already springing up to sell genetic analyses to the public.

Professor Topol had sent samples of his own DNA to a few companies and got back analyses that allegedly showed his susceptibility to different diseases. As a good scientist he tried to assess their methodologies before he was prepared to trust their results. He concluded from what he could learn about their methods was that they were a very mixed bag. Some appeared to be rigorous in their methodologies, others looked very dubious and even claimed to be able to do things he knew that they couldn't.

In any case what do you do now, he wondered aloud, if you know that the likelihood of your having high blood pressure is, say, 28% greater than the average and your chance of type 2 diabetes is 17% less? Perhaps, he mused, it might motivate him to change his lifestyle a bit; but there again, maybe it wouldn't.

Some of his fellow Americans had other answers. He showed us copies of Lonely Hearts advert where men specified that they wanted to meet women without the variants on the *BRCA1* and *BRCA2* genes that were linked with breast cancer. Others offered to supply details of their own genome as evidence of their desirability. One company offered a gene matching dating service to the general public. We were watching as a new industry was born.

We have challenges and we have choices

This chapter explores some of the ways we can use science – how we can apply the knowledge it generates and what sort of systems we need to put in place if its findings are to have the biggest impact on our health.

Scientific discoveries, as scientists know only too well, can be used for good or bad purposes. This chapter looks at how science and systems can help to create greater independence and better health for all. There is a danger, however, that they may be used to create greater dependence and to benefit only the more wealthy and powerful.

We must face up to three challenges if we are to succeed in creating greater independence and better health for all. I have called these the challenges of 'early health, independence and equity'.

The first, the *early health* challenge, is that we currently spend enormous sums of money on treating illness, much more than we spend on preventing it. Our whole system is geared towards treatment. Most health companies and professionals make their living from treating our illnesses rather than from preventing them. How can we use the new discoveries of science and the new technologies to give more attention to prevention of disease and the promotion of health?

Far more information is available to us as individuals now than ever before, thanks to the Internet and the power of technology; but it is also much harder to tell what is accurate and relevant and to know what sources and sites to trust. Our second *independence* challenge is how to ensure that this increase in information genuinely promotes greater patient control and independence. Or will it only increase our dependence on the professionals to interpret for us what it all means?

The third *equity* challenge is the simplest to state, but the hardest to deal with. Can we make sure that the African, Asian or South American mother in a poor rural village is able to give her children the healthcare, vaccines and treatments they need? Will the poorest people in richer countries get the science and the care they need?

We have choices about what we do (Figure 8.1).

Professor Topol's lecture brought out very well the challenges and choices we face in the use of new scientific discovery. It also revealed something of the complexities that surround them. There are profound ethical and political issues here about stem cell research, abortion and about using 'hybrid' embryos as well as about how far we want to see equity in the world and a sharing of the benefits of human endeavour.

```
┌─────────────────────────────────────────────────────┐
│                                                       │
│         We can choose to pursue:                      │
│                                                       │
│      •   Early health or late disease                 │
│                                                       │
│      •   Independence or dependence                   │
│                                                       │
│      •   Equity or inequality                         │
│                                                       │
└─────────────────────────────────────────────────────┘
```

Figure 8.1 Three choices about how we make use of science

There are also great risks both in the science itself and in the access to knowledge. These new scientific techniques may create new problems, the unexpected and unintended consequences of progress. Will we see new diseases and conditions created and will scientists in relieving human beings of one disease, create people who are much more vulnerable to others?

Will greater access to knowledge by the public also cause problems? Will people act entirely without the influence and guidance of the professionals? Will they, as so many parents did with regard to MMR in the UK, decide they know better?

Early health

There are many ways in which this science can help us move upstream to address our first early health challenge of giving greater emphasis to the prevention of disease and promotion of health. Here I describe briefly a few examples of the areas where genetics, better diagnostics and the better understanding of child and embryo development can all bring great benefits.

Genetic analysis has already led to big improvements in pre-natal screening and the ability, controversial as it is, to choose embryos without the mutations on certain genes that are known to be associated with specific diseases or to have the foetuses treated in utero. Some couples where one or both partners carry high genetic risks of particular conditions or diseases are also now having themselves screened and, depending on the results, deciding not to have children or planning a careful programme of screening for every pregnancy.

Genetic screening is even being used routinely by at least one whole group of people for pre-marital testing to identify the risks faced by any children of their marriages. The Ashkenazi Jews of New York have over the centuries intermarried within a relatively small population. As a result there is a higher than average number of similar mutations on genes and a greater risk of congenital conditions and pre-dispositions to particular diseases. They now routinely arrange genetic screening before marriage.

In other applications of this science, gene therapy, although itself in its infancy, is used to replace genes at a later stage of life with a particular mutation known to be associated with a disease with others that don't carry the same risk.

Early health is not just about genetics. Professor Topol is based at the Scripps Institute in San Diego. Further up on the west coast of the USA, Professor Lee Hartwell, President of the Fred Hutchinson Cancer Centre in Seattle, has, together with Jeff Trent and

George Posle, created the Partnership for Personalized Medicine. It is now part of the Centre for Sustainable Health, founded by Lee with Dr. Michael Birt.

Professor Hartwell has a vision for the Partnership that goes way beyond the purely academic. He is a great scientist; with a Nobel Prize for his work on the fundamental processes that underlie cell division. He is very far, however, from the caricature of the unworldly professor, who is focussed only on his science and the life of the mind.

He is passionate about the use and application of his science in the real world and its potential benefit to society. He is interested in practical knowledge. His aim for the Partnership is that it should develop biological tests that would enable early diagnosis of disease and in turn allow for early treatment. They would not only improve health outcomes but also and importantly, he stresses the 'importantly', reduce health care costs.

He points to the extraordinary growth in healthcare costs in his own country and to the fact that early treatment is much less expensive. Treatment of advanced-stage cancer may typically be five or more times higher than for early stage, with of course a far worse prognosis for the patient and far more pain and suffering in the meantime.

The facts are, as Professor Hartwell says, indisputable. The cost of treating cervical cancer at an early 'localised' stage was around US$20 000, whilst the cost of treating late-stage cancer that had spread was nearer US$100 000 in the USA in the early 1990s. Patients had a better than 90% chance of surviving for 5 years with a localised cancer, but a worse than 20% chance for one that had spread.[2]

The science is now at the point, Professor Hartwell believes, when it is possible to develop a very wide range of potential diagnostic tests very quickly and relatively cheaply. The Partnership brings together health insurers, service providers, clinicians and researchers so that they can trial the tests within the populations they serve, testing out both their efficacy and their application.[2]

There are also scientists working on this in poorer countries. There are vaccine development programmes underway in the most common communicable diseases. PATH, for example, also based in Seattle, is supported by the Gates Foundation to develop new diagnostics as well as other technologies for use in poor countries. In the UK Dr Helen Lee of Cambridge University has an extensive programme of developing simple and inexpensive technologies suitable for use in making diagnoses in the environment and conditions of poor countries.[3]

In talking of early health, not late disease I have borrowed the phrasing used by Sir Bill Castell, the then Chairman of GE Healthcare, at the Pacific Health Conference in 2005 when he talked about how the power of "biology, bytes and broadband" had the potential to change the whole way medicine was managed by early diagnosis and treatment.[4] He argued that we were now developing the technology that would allow us to analyse tissues and samples so quickly and so effectively that we could diagnose diseases early and be able to develop early treatments or, better still, take evasive action, and avoid the disease altogether. We could start to design-in health to our bodies; we wouldn't be in the position, as we are now, where we have to respond to diseases.

If Sir Bill and others are right, the introduction of these technologies will require a complete re-thinking of the way health systems work. Logically we should pour our resources into prevention, promotion and early diagnosis and we should be able, over time, to reduce our investment in tackling late disease.

It is the dream that so many people working in public health have been following for so long. They argue that, even without the new science, we should have been putting the greater part of our efforts into health promotion and disease prevention for years.

We are already, of course, paying increasing attention in rich countries to reducing smoking, improving diet and taking exercise and accompanying this with education, population screening, immunisation, improvements in the environment and, in some cases, the treatment of whole populations with vitamins, food supplements and fluoride. In rich countries many of us are taking drugs such as statins and angiotensin-converting enzyme (ACE) inhibitors prophylactically to ward off later disease.

We are also just beginning to understand the implications of the work of Dr David Barker, referred to in Chapter 2, who has shown that what happens before birth profoundly influences our life chances thereafter. Adequate and appropriate nutrition and care in 'the world within our mothers' dramatically improves our health because as he puts it 'heart attacks begin in the womb'.[5]

As we have seen earlier, we are still in general wedded to an expensive healthcare model where we concentrate on late treatment. It seems like an almost impossibly big task to re-design the entire system around prevention and promotion. The current incentives are against us, there is enormous inertia and there would, undoubtedly, be concerted and powerful pushback. How and where could you get leverage to turn this all upside down?

These developments, however, suggest that there is some hope that we could look to science, which has so long been associated with the development of new and ever more expensive high-tech treatments, to play a bigger role in *early health*. Scientific discovery could be much more focussed on the tests and interventions of early diagnosis and not just on the drugs and treatments of late disease.

We need treatments for later disease. Not everything will be prevented or be preventable, but we need to invest heavily in the scientific potential to boost early diagnosis and intervention. We need to make this a priority even though it goes against all the current incentives in the system and the training and experience of the professionals. Policymakers and scientists have a real choice to make.

Promoting independence

Science and technology can also play a major role in helping us to live our lives as independently as we wish, with greater personal control at every stage. Again, a few examples illustrate just some of the potential.

The work of scientists like Professor Topol opens up the possibilities of so-called 'personalised medicine', where drugs and therapies can be targeted on, and even designed for, a specific patient. We already know that particular drugs for hypertension, for example, only work for that part of the population who have a particular mutation on a specific gene. If clinicians know which people have the mutation they can use this knowledge to prescribe accurately for those people and not waste the drug on others where it will be ineffective.

Genetic analysis at the individual level will allow us as patients to discuss our health and possible treatments in a much more detailed way than ever before, with a sharing of information and decision making.

These scientific advances are already helping to change the relationship between patients and professionals, as envisaged in our second 'independence' challenge. As individuals we can use the Internet, have direct access to the science and the scientists and diagnose ourselves. They can remove the need for the mediator and reinforce control by the patient.

We also see this happening with the development of new technologies that allow us to monitor and manage our own health and healthy behaviour. There is the phone that photographs our plates before and after we have eaten from them and estimates our calorific intake, the implanted devices that continuously monitor our vital signs and can send messages back to our doctors and the many ways in which we ourselves can be alerted to problems or simply reminded that we should take our medication.

There are now systems that bring together all the information we might want to know about our food intake, sleep patterns, exercise and vital signs and report back to us on our overall health. Some of them can even get our personal physician on a video link if we breach any of the parameters we have set.

Everywhere we go our whole life can be monitored and assessed. Our personal electronic health record will be available day and night to record not only the care we have been given but also every test and analysis we have chosen to put ourselves through. Everywhere we go we can plan: with Internet access to the health value of individual items on restaurant menus and to the amounts of energy we will exert and the exercise we will get by different sorts of activity. Technology can help us take control.

Businesses are already designing products that allow us not just to monitor ourselves, but also to ensure that our elderly parents are taking their pills, eating, sleeping and in reasonable health. If they aren't, these systems, probably run through our phones, will alert us and the local health system. This may not just be a better way of doing things; it may also be cheaper than current models of care. Our elderly parents, of course, may object to this electronic tagging and surveillance and prefer that we don't know so much about what they are up to!

The joggers and runners we see today with their heart rate monitors strapped to their arms and their pedometers counting their steps, their speed and their expenditure of energy, will also have a dream come true. Programming, planning and reviewing: they will be in total control every step of the way. These patients know it and want it.

Another group that are benefiting from the continuing progress of science and technology are people with disabilities who are able to get back some of their functionality and therefore their independence through better prostheses, aids and the developing ability to manipulate mechanical devices with brain power as well as muscles. At a larger scale, the development of all the spare part surgery and particularly the now routine replacements of hips, knees and lenses, has allowed a generation of people much more mobility and independence than their parents ever had.

The scope for improving our independence seems almost limitless.

Equity

These examples, some already with us and some merely promises to come, all show how science and technology used in this way can offer greater independence and better health.

However, they all require money and almost all also require the ability and confidence of the patients to handle the knowledge and engage with their clinicians.

For many people, less affluent and educated, they may simply serve to increase differences between rich and poor, the 'haves' and 'have nots', and serve to increase dependence – both within a country and internationally. The access that people have to these advances will depend on the availability of resources, on how health services and systems are organised and on the myriad social, cultural and political issues, which we have seen in earlier chapters influence health and healthcare.

The themes of early health, independence and equity resonate in poorer countries. Early health and the establishment of local health programmes with the emphasis on immunisation, clean water, mosquito bed nets and the education of women are central to health plans.

Independence fits very naturally into the environment of poor countries, where government health plans are generally part of the country's wider plans for social and economic development. Among non-governmental groups, the people of the Thar Desert in Rajasthan talk explicitly of self-determination as being the goal of their economic, social and health programmes. BRAC in Bangladesh and others use very similar language.

Health and development can go hand in hand, the one reinforcing the other. Better health means that potentially there is a healthier and more productive working population. Progress in development, with better education and more money, can mean that the population becomes healthier.

Whilst equity, with a focus on getting at least basic health services to all parts of a population may be an aspiration for many, the reality is often very different. It is not just that the local elite live very differently from most of the people in the country, but that remote and rural populations fare worse than most urban ones and the poorest in all populations worst of all.

A major part of the problem here, as elsewhere, is how to find the resources necessary and how to make them reach the poorest. There is a need within countries to create the right incentives and many have been experimenting with schemes to offer financial and other rewards to health workers who will stay in the most remote areas and work with the poorest people. Some are also trying, as President Obama is doing in the USA, to extend insurance schemes to the poorest.

International organisations, recognising that private companies have no incentives to create products for the poorest countries and populations, have created the International Financing Facility for Immunization[6] and the Advanced Market Commitment to fund the development of vaccines and drugs for the major communicable diseases that mainly only affect poor countries. In treating TB, as shown earlier, clinicians have not had a new diagnostic test for 100 years or a new drug for 40. This scheme creates a viable business model for pharmaceutical, biotech and other companies to invest in the long and expensive period of research and development.

In 2009, the report of the Task Force on Innovative International Financing for Health Systems, chaired by the World Bank President and the British Prime Minister, proposed extending this sort of arrangement to other areas and advocated the creation of voluntary contributions from air travellers and others to creating the funding necessary to improve health systems and health. These proposals were accepted at a meeting of the UN in September 2009.[7]

At the same time prolonged campaigning has led to some commercial organisations changing their own internal business models so as to provide the same drug or product at cheaper prices in poorer countries. Some therapies are now much more widely available than they were.

Other businesses have been looking at how they, too, can operate in poorer countries. Craig Mundie, as befits the Technical Director of Microsoft, has written about the needs of poor countries in *Information Technology: Advancing Global Health*.[8] He believes that, with the enormous numbers of people wanting healthcare in poor countries, it will not be possible to have the same people-centred model of treatment and care as we have now in richer countries. We can't all go and see the doctor at once. He believes that we will have to make much more use of technology, using greater machine-to-machine interaction to reduce costs, cut out processes and reach remote areas.

In a small room at the conference centre in Seattle he showed me a mocked-up version of an icon-driven PC that could be used by an illiterate person to describe her child's illness. It had pictures of babies and adult men and women accompanied by symbols of parts of the body that allowed them to describe the problem in some detail. The data they entered was transmitted to another machine that arranged it according to protocols into a useable form and then, and only then, passed it to a far-distant clinician for attention.

This may not be immediately applicable today but one can sense something of the shape of the future here in Craig's insight that only through greater use of machines can we achieve the scale poor countries need at a cost they might be able to afford. Craig also told me how he saw this as a businessman. "At the moment", he said, "We only have around 1.7 billion customers and don't serve the other 4.9 billion or so". Of those 4.9 billion he believed about 3.9 billion had some element of disposable income and could, as they have done with mobile phones, buy technology if it were cheap enough. For the other billion he thought governments, national and international, would have to bear the cost of bringing them into the digital age.

The commercial point that some products can be made down to a price for people with a small disposable income but that government needs in some way to subsidise or pump prime investment for the poorest is crucial. It is part of the rationale for the International Financing Facility for Immunization scheme.

This discussion underscores the importance of the relationship between commercial interests in emerging markets and government action in developing countries in creating and using knowledge and in together helping lift the poor out of poverty.

Science and technology can help in very many ways. Mobile phones have provided an extraordinary boost in poor countries. Their widespread use allows farmers to phone ahead and decide which market is offering the best prices and traders to negotiate deals at a distance. Within health, mobile phones, the Internet and the power of microprocessors have opened up the opportunities to diagnose, advise and treat patients at a distance. Telemedicine in all its forms can make a huge difference in poor countries.[9]

These relationships are very important; technology and commercial interests have significant roles to play. Governments and the Gates Foundation are investing heavily in developing the technology that is needed. However, this is only one part of the equation; we need to know how to apply the knowledge and the technology to best effect.

Applying what we know today

This is the fourth challenge that we must face in making best use of science and technology: the challenge of applying the knowledge we have. We may have the knowledge and technology we want and we may know how we want to use it, but do we actually know how to apply it in practice? Do we have the practical knowledge of what to do in reality? This is not as easy as it may seem.

Over 1.5 million children die every year in poor countries from dehydration caused by diarrhoea.[10] Most of their deaths could be prevented.[11] More than 90% of blind people live in poor countries; 75% of blindness is avoidable or treatable.[12] We know what needs to be done. In the USA, as we saw in Chapter 3, half of all the care that is given is suboptimal and doesn't follow available evidence and known good practice. We very often fail to apply the knowledge we have.

As Pang et al, writing in *The Lancet*, assert: "Applying what we know already will have a bigger impact in health and disease than any drug or technology likely to be introduced in the next decade."[13]

This is not just a problem for poor countries nor is it just about resources. New discoveries may take years to become widely used by clinicians. It took 20 years before clot-busting drugs were routinely given immediately after heart attacks in the UK. The irony was that when they were finally normal practice everywhere, research had shown that direct-access angioplasty was a more effective therapy. The work of spreading knowledge and practice had to start all over again. Even today, as four eminent clinicians write in the New York Times, there is an enormous divide between hospitals providing high cost low quality care and those providing low cost high quality care in the United States. Knowledge simply isn't being applied and spread.[14]

Part of the problem is to do with the cultural, social and political factors that we discussed in the last chapter and all of which can help or hinder the application of technology and knowledge. We need to link the outputs of the natural sciences with the social sciences so as to understand how things get done in practice and what role patients, the public and society as a whole play alongside scientists and clinicians.

Part, too, is due to internal health and system-related issues. Applying knowledge within a health system can be very complex because it involves decisions made by thousands of individual clinicians and millions of patients and may involve re-training, changing clinical practices and systems as well as overcoming cultural and social barriers.[15,16]

This single example of clot-busting drugs in the NHS shows how important it is to learn how to apply the knowledge we have as quickly as possible. The NHS has the advantage of being an integrated and organised health system. Applying knowledge in the environment of poor countries can be even more difficult with the natural barriers of distance and scattered communities and the low level of resources, let alone the absence in many places of anything resembling a health system.

Strengthening health systems

As I write this in 2009 'strengthening health systems' has become one of the major objectives of international development and health. The World Health Organization (WHO) and other influential bodies have recognised that we can't apply the knowledge we have without a functioning health system in place within a country and international efforts to increase health funding are concentrating on strengthening systems and on re-emphasising the important role of national leadership.[7]

For some years the organisations running the Global Health Initiatives, such as the Global Fund, President's Emergency Fund for AIDS (PEPFAR) and Global Action on Vaccination and Immunization (GAVI), were able to operate by setting up their own project management and delivery systems and ignoring wider health issues in a country. It was the fastest and most efficient way to deliver their services, but, as described in Chapter 5, had some downsides including the fact that national leadership and national health systems were often sidelined or even weakened.

Thinking has moved on, lessons have been learned and there is now a great deal of activity internationally designed to bring together efforts at strengthening systems with the Global Health Initiatives and creating new ways of working that strengthen national systems and leadership whilst delivering on the specific goals.

The WHO has described system strengthening as being about six elements - service delivery, financing, governance, health workforce, information systems and supply management systems – and at a conference in mid-2009 has started to design how these things may be done in practice with the active participation of the Global Health Initiatives.[17] These developments seem to herald a new era in development approaches to health.

The risks in system strengthening

These developments, together with the renewed commitments to additional funding, are enormously positive and show how much the international community has learned from the past and is determined to create a new approach.

There is still a lot of thinking to do, however, and some very practical questions to be asked about how best to implement the new approach, how to ensure the new investment is used most effectively and how to make sure that the knowledge we have about what works is available everywhere. The organisations involved are very aware of the need for good implementation processes and, in the words of the Task Force on Innovative Financing, "How to get more funding for health and more health for the funding".

There is an obvious danger that implementation might concentrate on building capacity and not on how that capacity is used. Both are needed. At its worst a small and poorly functioning health system will be replaced by a larger and equally poorly functioning one. There is a lot of work underway on productivity, target setting, gaining community buy-in, strengthening national leadership and other important aspects. But there are other dangers too.

We faced them in the NHS in 2000 when we set ourselves short-term input targets for increases in doctors and nurses and longer term targets for outcomes, such as the reduction in deaths from coronary heart diseases. We were very conscious of the risk that we would concentrate more on the short-term building up of capacity than on the longer term improvements and, accordingly, set up the Modernisation Agency as an internal change agent to help improve our practices and use the new money and the new staff to best effect.

We were successful, but there were difficulties. These were partly because of the different timescales and the fact that we knew how to recruit staff and could do so quickly whilst we were still learning how best to change our practices to deliver the outcomes. The other part of the reason, which is also very relevant to this discussion, was that there was public and political pressure to see fast results. We were able to show them the rapidly increasing staff numbers; service transformation took longer.

There are two dangers for poor countries inherent in this story. The first is that they will build the capacity of the existing system and then have to retrain staff and develop new practices.

The second danger is that they will import practices from rich countries that simply don't fit. This will be very tempting because it will take less time and seem easier to import existing practices rather than create new ones. Moreover, as they will be receiving lots of advice from richer countries, it will be very easy unconsciously to adopt the ideas and ideologies that accompany the money and the scientific knowledge.

Public and political pressure at home and abroad will demand quick improvements. Some can be made – there are quick wins – but others will take a great deal of time.

These problems highlight the need for a sophisticated and well thought through approach to implementation and draw out an aspect that appears, so far, to be being largely ignored in the international debates about implementation – how systematically to improve clinical practices and services in ways suitable to the local context and environment. The cultural, social and political aspects of health and healthcare discussed in the last chapter are very relevant here.

This is fundamental. Many existing services are very poor, many staff are poorly trained and supervised and many practices are out of date or inappropriate. Changes will be needed and a successful implementation methodology needs to have improvement at its heart.

Implementing improvement

Effective implementation starts with a good understanding of how systems function in health and elsewhere. At its simplest a health system can be viewed as made up of a number of parts – such as patients and health workers, facilities and equipment, governance arrangements, processes and subsystems – which work together to perform a function. Changing one part by, say, introducing new equipment or providing new information to patients will affect every other part in some way.

Successful implementation takes account of these simple insights. Successful implementers need the practical knowledge of how to do so. Don Berwick, the charismatic President of the Institute for Healthcare Improvement (IHI), puts it very simply:

"Our approach to quality improvement views healthcare as a large, complex system of interdependent actors (patients, care providers, payers, policymakers) and organisations

(hospitals, primary care, public health entities, communities). This approach views performance as an inherent property of the system, linked inevitably to its design. Just as the top speed of a car is a property of that car, the waiting times in a healthcare organisation or the maternal death rates in a community are properties of that organisation and that community as they are currently designed.

From this viewpoint, all improvement requires change to existing processes. Simply stressing or exhorting current systems to 'do better' will not yield fundamentally different results. Changing those systems may."[18]

The IHI has over the last 20 years established an international reputation for quality improvement in health and for 'spreading good practice'. It does precisely what its name says it does: healthcare improvement. In the Institute's own words:

"*The Institute helps accelerate change in healthcare by cultivating promising concepts for improving patient care and turning those ideas into action*".[19]

It does so by applying and developing the quality improvement methods developed over years in other industries through the work of people like Demming, Juran, Feigenbaum and others to healthcare.

The IHI has an inspirational leadership team led by Professor Don Berwick and Maureen Bisognano. Both are experienced clinicians – Don is Clinical Professor of Paediatrics at Harvard and Maureen is a nurse and former Hospital Chief Executive – who are grounded in the day-to-day reality of providing healthcare. They founded the Institute because they were so concerned about the quality failures in the American health system and saw the potential of thinking in terms of system and of systematically making change.

Where health planners typically start with the big picture of what needs doing and work downwards, Don, Maureen and colleagues start at the local level with the actual clinical practice and work up. Where health planners may typically try to solve the whole problem in one go by thinking through all the aspects and producing a master plan for success, Don and Maureen will more likely start by looking at the detail, understanding how the local system works and what influences it, changing a part, seeing what happens and changing something else. They deal in the practical reality of clinical practice. They turn the world upside down.

In a recent example of their work, the IHI took some ideas about how using a 'bundle' of therapies in intensive care might be more effective than the traditional single or sequential use, tested this in a number of clinical locations to ensure that it really was good practice, identified the circumstances under which it worked and then took it to scale as part of its 100,000 Lives Campaign.[20,21]

This campaign set out with the very ambitious goal of avoiding 100000 unnecessary deaths in American hospitals in the 18 months from January 2005 to June 2006. It worked by identifying the conditions needed for success. These included such expected factors as leadership commitment within hospitals, having clear aims and creating a system for measuring progress. They also included identifying and packaging proven ideas and practices and creating a process for refining the plan in response to learning during implementation.

The Campaign chose six proven interventions that would have a high impact on the quality of care and the survival of patients. These ranged from preventing central line infections to drug reconciliation and preventing ventilator-associated pneumonia. It worked by supporting hospitals throughout the USA to learn the improvement methodologies and implement improvements in practice. In each case a team in the hospital worked through what it needed to do locally to create the right conditions and implement known best practice.

A core part of the methodology is the **P**lan **D**o **S**tudy **A**ct (PDSA) cycle (Figure 8.2) through which teams planned a change that they thought might help, implemented it, studied the result and acted on what was learned. They **p**lanned, **d**id, **s**tudied and **a**cted. All this was done as quickly as possible with one change following another as they cumulatively improved practice and outcomes. As part of the Campaign they shared ideas and experiences with other hospitals and were able to learn from their PDSA cycles and their successes and failures as well as from their own.

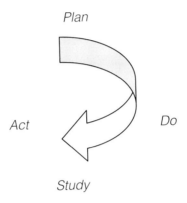

Figure 8.2 The PDSA cycle

I saw this cycle used in the NHS when we decided that we would improve treatment and treatment times in our Accident and Emergency Departments (or Emergency Rooms) and ensure that nobody waited more than 4 hours to be treated or admitted to hospital. We brought hospitals together in groups and worked with them as they designed improvements.

One hospital might decide, for example, that treatment times would be improved if nurses could order X-rays and not have to wait for a doctor to do so. Another turned the whole system upside down by deciding that it might do better if the most senior person saw patients first, because they were better able to make quick and accurate decisions. A third introduced near-patient pathology tests, thus cutting out the waiting time for results to come back from a distant laboratory. Within 6 weeks they had seen the results and were also able to learn from what happened in the other hospitals. They repeated the PDSA cycle with another change and so on, as they searched for improvement.

We succeeded. By 2005 every hospital was achieving 98% of patients treated or admitted within 4 hours, with this improvement maintained today. In each case the solution was designed by local people to address local conditions. The evidence they were using in every case was the same, but the solution was not.

Returning to the USA, The 100 000 Lives Campaign had a major impact on improvement in US hospitals – the participating hospitals avoided about 120 000 deaths in the 18 month period, although this cannot be attributed to the campaign alone.[21]

It is a spectacular result achieved by changing the way systems function and people work, with little or no additional resources. Joe McCannon, the IHI Vice President who led the campaign explained to me that each of their 200 mentor hospitals - which had been asked to produce exemplar practice - succeeded in introducing better practice in very different ways. He went on to say:

"Precisely because IHI has no formal power to enforce clinical guidelines, we cannot mandate that change happen in a particular way. Instead we generate ideas and will by learning what is happening at the front lines in the most agile way possible and shining a light on successes. Often other hospitals will find ideas in the success of these mentors though when they invent something themselves, we also need to capture that and celebrate them so others will seek their coaching.

The same applies across all of our work and the core skill, which everything in western pedagogy and training seems to oppose, is not to teach but to learn what is happening in other places as quickly as possible and redistribute it rapidly. The role of the NGO or government, then, is not to lead hierarchical change but to manage an ecosystem of random learning events and make knowledge available fast.

An important, related skill becomes managing dissemination in such a way that it yields results - I think there is a need to think about this as a new science that the world needs to learn."

Over the years the IHI has developed and refined its approaches so that it is now able to teach people how to improve quality with the aid of well-tested approaches and techniques. In response to demand from medical students it has now established the IHI Open School, which provides free access to its ideas and approaches to thousands of students and others.

The IHI's ideas and methodologies are now being spread and used around the world. We learned a great deal from them in the UK and, for example, set up a coronary heart disease collaborative in 2002 to help identify and spread the good practice we needed to deliver the improvements in access to clot-busting drugs mentioned earlier. A year later, again influenced by the IHI, we published *10 High Impact Changes*, detailing the most effective and cost-effective interventions we had shown were necessary to improve the NHS.[23]

"Rich countries may be able to tolerate waste in their health systems, poor countries can't. Quality matters even more in poor countries"

These methods are beginning to be used more extensively in poorer countries, where cultural issues mean that it is perhaps even more important that local people design solutions locally.

They are used by the University Research Co (URC), funded by the United States Agency for International Development (USAID), in its development work in many poorer countries and the Pan American Organisation for Health (PAHO), the regional organisation of the WHO, has adopted them as their core methodology in reducing maternal mortality in the region. The IHI itself has also set up programmes in the last 5 years in South Africa, Malawi and Ghana.

There are difficulties, however, which we have identified before in using methods and practices from rich countries in poor ones. The IHI's work was developed in the very specific circumstances of the USA, where there are plenty of resources, where government plays a relatively small role and hospitals and service providers have dominated the environment. The IHI is learning in Africa how to work in very different circumstances, where the focus is on primary and community care and government is almost always a very big player.

Other countries have developed their own approach to improving quality. Dr Francis Omaswa, then the head of Medical service in the Ministry, set up an extensive quality improvement programme in Uganda in the late 1990s and helped found the South and East Africa Quality Centre at Makerere University, which is designed to help countries learn from each other. In Asia, the Public Health Foundation for India, has stated that one of its principal goals is to learn lessons in its environment for application in other middle- and low-income countries.

There is a great deal to be learned from the mixing of the different approaches to quality. In the autumn of 2008 a group of us, including Dr Omaswa and Professor Srinath Reddy, President of the Public Health Foundation for India, were brought together by the IHI and the Rockefeller Foundation to discuss whether and how to construct a framework for quality improvement in developing countries.

There were 22 people from 15 countries with a 50 : 50 split between developing and developed countries. Africa, India, Pakistan, China and South America were all represented, as were Europe and North America. Our numbers included ministers and ex-ministers, permanent secretaries and other civil servants, academics and representatives of voluntary organisations as well as faculty from the IHI; more than half were clinicians.

The reason we were there was because we knew about quality improvement in rich countries and had in *Crossing the Quality Chasm* a guide to the measurable dimensions of quality and a framework for action.[24] We suspected that this wouldn't be appropriate for developing countries and wondered if a different version would be needed. A literature survey carried out by Sheila Leatherman and Tim Ferris showed that we were starting with a clean sheet because there was very little systematic research about quality and improvement in developing countries and certainly no equivalent of this framework.

It seemed to all of us, from all our different perspectives, to be particularly important that, with increased amounts of money being spent on health in developing countries, there was some way of defining, assessing and improving quality.

The meeting was fascinating. It not only brought together two traditions but two sets of life experiences. We all liked the clean systematic science and logic of the IHI approach, but we were all very aware of the lack of resources and of the national and international politics that had to be managed in Africa, in particular, and developing countries in general. We had to find a way of combining the insights from both.

A framework like the one provided by *Crossing the Chasm* might be appropriate in a relatively well-ordered environment in the West but was irrelevant at this stage in poorer countries that were building their systems. What was needed much more immediately was a methodology to improve service at every step of the way.

We concluded that rather than developing a new framework at the moment, we should start from where we were and seek to ensure that existing policies in developing countries paid attention to quality. The big new theme in Africa was health systems strengthening, but, as we have also seen, it might be interpreted as being about capacity and not improvement, about quantity and not quality. We wanted to make sure that systems strengthening was about quality as well as quantity.

A quality improvement movement was born from that meeting that was designed around the African National Congress (ANC) slogan 'Awareness, Mobilisation, Organisation' so familiar to the South Africans in the room. We needed to raise awareness by demonstrating the success of the quality improvement methodologies and mobilise support and resources before being able to put in place the organisation needed to ensure that they were adopted everywhere. Our framework could only be designed towards the end of this process.

It was a very good example of how people from rich and poor countries could learn and work together. It was, to oversimplify, a meeting of American and European systems thinking and logic with African and Asian political thinking and pragmatic management. The result was the better for having both parties involved.

Whilst there were differences, more united us than separated us. There was a commitment to quality improvement and to continuously searching for ways to close the gap between what we aspired to and what we saw around us today. There was also a similar attitude to resources. Quality improvement is not about spending more money. It is about spending the money we have to the best effect.

As Francis Omaswa put it: "Rich countries may be able to tolerate waste in their health systems, poor countries can't. Quality matters even more in poor countries."

Protocols, guidelines and checklists

The account of this international meeting underlines the point that improving quality is not something that is done once only. Circumstances change, knowledge develops and new resources become available. All change the way systems work and all provide opportunities for improvement. Don Berwick argues strongly that all clinicians need to understand how to make improvement and to apply it continuously in their practice. He has demonstrated his own commitment by opening the IHI Open School but argues that all professional training should include training in improvement.

The same point about continuous improvement applies to the many guidelines, protocols and checklists that provide a very practical way for sharing knowledge. These show clinicians what steps to take in diagnosis and treatment for given symptoms or diseases.

Many such clinical protocols and guidelines have been developed over the years, so many indeed that clinicians have good reason to be confused about which ones to use and which to adhere to. For some, however, it is relatively easy because they work for an employer that specifies the treatment patients should receive and the protocols to follow.

At its worst this has been called 'cook book' medicine with the assertion that it is mindless medicine that reduces the doctor to a technician who need only follow instructions. Applying it ruthlessly, it was said, deprived clinicians of the right to make decisions and deprived patients of the best care. In some cases, perhaps where the clinician was too lazy or the payer too wedded to their protocol, this is bad for clinicians and patients.

Perhaps even worse, however, is that this sort of guideline can be used by the unscrupulous to direct clinicians to use a certain sort of drug or treatment to their commercial advantage. As always in medicine we need to ask cui bono? Often somebody does, other than the patient.

At its best, however, this is liberating medicine. It allows a clinician to see what is normal practice, what his or her peers believe works best, and to take a measured decision to follow this practice or do something different, if they think that is the right thing to do. As a patient it is comforting to know that a doctor knows what normal practice is and, if he or she decides to do something different, knows why they are doing so.

In 1995 Mike Stein, a young South African doctor working in Oxford, decided to create a software system that would enable clinicians to tap quickly into a comprehensive compendium of the best knowledge available at the time. He called it the Map of Medicine and designed it so that a clinician need only type in a symptom to locate a suitable protocol.

A doctor might for example type in 'stomach pain' and would immediately find themselves at the top of a decision tree that asked further questions about the precise location and nature and duration of the pain, guiding them gradually through their decision.

When Mike demonstrated it to me I was surprised to see that I could enter Homer Simpson as a starting point. This indicated that a patient had taken a drug known by this name, presumably because it turned you into an objectionable lunatic. It didn't matter that the clinician didn't know what drug a Homer Simpson actually was when the patient or his friend had told him he had taken one, as long as the software was up to date on the local usage.

Mike Stein designed and developed it within the NHS as part of our far-reaching information technology (IT) programme. It embraced the public interest values of the NHS by ensuring that the decision trees were written through a consensus of clinicians, none of whom were aligned with or paid by any commercial interests.

Most interestingly of all were two additional features that Mike incorporated from the start. At every stage in the decision process a clinician could find out what the evidence was that it was based on, simply by interrogating the software. This was updated regularly. Perhaps even more interesting is the fact that users can adapt the protocol themselves to fit their own circumstances. Thus, for example, a hospital might adapt the standard decision tree in The Map of Medicine on how to deal with a suspected deep vein thrombosis (DVT) to fit in with their own practice or to add detail about who to call or what facilities to use if a DVT is suspected.

The Map is a particularly good example of how knowledge can be systematically passed on and made available to a clinician as and when he or she needs it. It is the sort of mechanism that over time, as technology improves in poor countries, will help isolated clinicians even more than it helps those in US and UK health systems. As I write the WHO is considering using it to prepare decision trees for 20 diseases such as malaria that are common in Africa and to include in the protocol steps that are reasonable to take in the particular local environment.

Map of Medicine and others like it are important not only as useful vehicles for transferring and accessing knowledge, but also as providing a means for constantly improving practice and reflecting new learning. This account reminds us once again of the importance of localness: local design, local implementation and local understanding of the cultural, social, political and economic context and constraints. It also reminds us that, as Sir Michael Rawlins described so brilliantly in his Harveian Oration of 2006, the practical knowledge used by clinicians is contextual and current and requires the use of judgement.[25]

Strengthening health systems in poorer countries

A clearer picture of how to strengthen health systems in poorer countries is starting to emerge. It has at its heart national – and indeed provincial and more local – leadership and plans. International partners are developing longer term and more sustainable funding sources to provide support in a well-coordinated and coherent way to these national and local leaders. There is, in 2009, renewed energy and optimism.

The discussion in this chapter suggests that additionally there needs to be an implementation process that employs a systematic approach to improvement and quality and creates local solutions, designed by local people for the local cultural, social, physical and economic environment. The result of this combination is described in Figure 8.3.

All the global initiatives and organisations and the development partners supporting national leaders and their national plans to improve health and healthcare by strengthening health systems specifically in the areas of:

- *Service delivery*

- *Financing*

- *Governance*

- *Health workforce*

- *Information systems*

- *Supply management*

Coupled with increased and sustainable funding and better use of funding. Supported by an implementation process that employs a systematic approach to improvement and quality and creates local solutions, designed by local people for the local cultural, social, physical and economic environment.

Figure 8.3 Strengthening health systems in poorer countries

All this activity is currently focused on achieving the Millennium Development Goals and making progress towards the underlying vision of health for all. The independence to live a life that one has reason to value has not yet appeared as an ultimate goal.

Strengthening health systems in richer countries – retrofitting improvement

The priority in poorer countries is to strengthen, and sometimes establish for the first time, functioning health systems. There is often relatively little in the way of existing arrangements that might get in the way. The position in richer countries is very different. There are already well-established health systems, with their own ways of doing things, their own dynamics and their own vested interests that are likely to oppose change.

In some ways the poorer countries have an advantage over the USA, the UK and other richer countries when it comes to building health systems based on early health, the independence of their citizens and equity. There is less baggage to contend with. In these richer countries, however, the task is to retrofit changes into an existing and very strong system.

Here we look at two models that are being created in the country with the most complex and expensive health system of them all, the USA. Whilst President Obama is working from the outside to make the existing system function better by reforming insurance and extending coverage, these examples get inside the system and try to change systems, processes and behaviours from the inside out.

Professor Lee Hartwell established the Partnership for Personalized Medicine to begin the development of a new system within the USA that would, amongst other things, support the introduction of early diagnostics. The Partnership is structured in an innovative way. It is a non-profit initiative; because as he says, in an echo of earlier discussions:

"Current economic incentives assure that companies will develop the most expensive new therapeutics and devices while neglecting the power of new diagnostics to improve health at reduced cost."[2]

It is the very antithesis of the new businesses that Professor Topol described so amusingly that are now springing up to exploit the new genetic discoveries. Where they are for private profit, it is for public good. Where they are about packaging products for markets, it is about creating new products through rigorous science. Where they are exclusive, it is inclusive.

Left to their own devices, Lee Hartwell suggests, private businesses have the incentive to look for the most profitable developments and applications in early diagnosis precisely as they do with late disease. Left alone, early diagnosis could become just as expensive, with companies filing patents and levying high prices. There will be a 'biological divide' just as there is a 'digital divide' where the best science is available to the rich and not the poor.

Professor Hartwell's ingenious non-profit partnership model, however, goes about this quite differently. He wants to work with healthcare payers, the insurance and mutual organisations who have an incentive to keep costs low, to identify the areas where new diagnostic tests would be most effective and cost effective. He is interested in the most effective and not the most profitable.

Once these areas are identified he wants the scientists in the partnership to work on developing the tests and, once potential tests are identified, he wants the clinicians and health care providers in the partnership to test them out in their populations. The Hartwell approach is only just being put into practice. It remains to be tested by reality. It embodies, however, a number of principles; all of which are important in understanding how knowledge can be applied effectively in the field of health.

It brings together many partners with different perspectives and different skills in a joint effort. They are all, clinicians, scientists, executives and business people involved in bringing about change and owning its success. It engages public and private sector interests, not one without the other. There are enough people with a stake in the venture to make this a powerful enough combination to begin to challenge the status quo. It is showing how it is possible to start to build a health system around early health.

Very interestingly, it also introduces an incentive for all the partners to start to think about the populations they serve. Typically, in the USA and many other countries the emphasis of healthcare providers and clinicians has been on taking care of individual patients or patient groups. Here all the partners need to think about the whole population they serve if the diagnostic tests are to be tested out. It shifts thinking towards a population base. Once we begin to think in terms of populations and not just patients, it is easier to begin to think about how to make sure that the benefits of the new science can be shared more evenly within the population, whether it is the population of Seattle or of the whole world.

The new sciences, applied in the way that Professor Harwell has outlined, could be a powerful new factor that might help tip the balance in favour of early health, independence and equity within the USA.

As radical as the new biology

In another departure from the mainstream, IHI is developing a programme called the Triple Aim with partners in North America and Europe to try to understand what a system that really improved health would look like.

The whole programme is based on the very simple insight that the key question for any health system is how to get the right balance between three desirable health care aims: improving individual experience, improving population health and controlling per capita cost.

No one or two of the aims are good enough by themselves; all three are necessary. As citizens, we definitely want all three. However, as Tom Nolan, one of the founders of the programme says speaking of his own country: "The root of the problem in health care is that the business models of almost all US health care organisations depend on keeping these three aims separate. Society on the other hand needs these three aims optimised (given appropriate weightings on the components) simultaneously."

It is a very simple and obvious idea, yet it challenges many of the assumptions and practices of western medicine and could change the way clinicians and organisations work. It could, if implemented, turn our world upside down.

Tom Nolan is one of a group of four people who used to work as statisticians in the US Agriculture Service but now run their own company, Associates in Performance Improvement (API), which has over the years become more and more involved in healthcare. They have formed a strong partnership with the IHI, bringing statistical rigour and insight to the IHI's knowledge of health and their focus on quality improvement and systems thinking. It is a powerful combination.

Triple Aim has been set up as a typical IHI/API research and development project. It tests out ideas at the most local level with people actually working on the problem, builds a prototype based on this experience and tests it again before going to scale. The goal, as always with IHI, is to find out what works and then spread the good practice. Equipped with their initial ideas about Triple Aim, Tom Nolan and John Whittington, a very experienced family physician, recruited around a dozen organisations from across the USA to join them in working through the ideas in practice. They are trying to identify the central features of Triple Aim organisations.

As I write Triple Aim has been under development for 2 years. Organisations from Canada, the UK and Sweden have joined the programme to help with the prototyping, bringing a rich mix of experience and skill to the enterprise. All the participants are finding the experience challenging, bringing into question as it does some of their most basic assumptions about how their own system operated.

The North American participants have the particular difficulty of working in systems that simply don't share the three aims. Generally American hospitals focus on providing services for their insured and paid-up populations and on making sure that their revenues grow. It is not normal American practice for hospitals to want to reduce costs or to be concerned about the local population who are not their patients. They have the one aim and ignore the other two.

The Primary Care Trusts from England's NHS that have joined the project are much more naturally suited to Triple Aim as the NHS embodies the aims of personal care and population health and works within a budget. However, even they are challenged about the balances between the three aims and face the same problem of a powerful system where all the incentives favour giving the most attention to the aim of personal care.

There is also a great deal of common ground. Discussions have frequently concentrated on the fact that, as we saw in Chapter 3, it is a relatively small group of patients who account for most of the costs of healthcare. Many people throughout the rich countries of the world are pursuing the goal of caring for people in their community, dealing with their social as well as health needs and avoiding the costs and discomforts of hospital. Triple Aim's unique contribution, however, is that it brings population, the individual and costs together and tries to understand how pursuing these three aims at once would work in practice.

They are testing out with their collaborators what pursuing Triple Aim would mean in reality for patients and families, for clinicians and for the teams delivering care, for the organisations working in health care and, ultimately, for health systems and whole societies. It is systematic search to understand the implications and to refine the concepts.

Through Triple Aim, the IHI and API are creating a part of the new knowledge we need. They are beginning to help us see what a new system might look like. There is a hopeful sense of a new way of approaching healthcare being developed and a gathering of momentum. Triple Aim is potentially as radical in its application and implications as the new biology we discussed earlier.

Private companies and public benefit; government and innovation

These last discussions have once again shown how private businesses, governments, NGOs and social enterprises all play significant roles in health and healthcare. They often work in partnership with each other and, increasingly, within large-scale and complex groupings and alliances. The relationships and boundaries between them all are shifting as people search for ever more effective ways of delivering services and working with patients and the public.

We have explored briefly the world of social enterprises, which use business methods for social ends, and touched on the many roles that different NGOs play from service provision to education and advocacy. Here we look in more detail at the relationships between private enterprises and government.

Commercial endeavour, as we saw earlier, is a very powerful part of the western scientific medicine paradigm. Linked with science and professionalism it has driven both innovation and costs. Increasingly, however, it is becoming constrained by regulation, by its position as a customer of government and by public opinion.

Whilst regulation is well established in richer countries, and overburdensome in some cases, it is very underdeveloped and even absent in many poorer ones. The fact that it is the poorest people who are most likely to be cheated, given counterfeit drugs or dangerous treatments has led even the staunchly business-orientated World Economic Forum to argue that the most important role for government in these poorer countries is to regulate healthcare so as to drive up quality and drive the quacks and cheats out of business.[26]

At the global level, regulation is much more complex because it involves so many different countries and authorities and because we enter into value-based arguments about what value we place on public goods as opposed to private ones. This is well illustrated by the continuing debates about the ownership and patenting of genetic material, where commercial interests patent our genes and scientists from the rich world go 'bio-prospecting' for genetic material amongst the diverse populations of the poor countries. Having secured the intellectual property, these organisations can sell or licence access to it, arguing that their creativity and hard work has created its value. Thousands of patents on human DNA have been filed and granted in this way.

Many people oppose this patenting. Professor Sir David Weatherall and his colleagues described the problem in the *Report on Genomics and World Health* produced for the WHO and they, like others, have argued that the monopolies awarded to commercial organisations by allowing them to patent genes are not in the public interest.[27]

As I write, the tangled issues around patenting human material and the wider aspects of intellectual property remain largely unresolved. In 2006 Indonesia, a very large middle-income country, took a stand on the related issue of rich countries benefiting from the human tissue of poor populations. It refused to release tissue from avian flu victims to WHO scientists. It reasoned that the material would be used to help create vaccines, which, because of costs, would only be available to people in rich countries. It wanted a share in any vaccines produced so that its population could benefit.

There can hardly be a more important issue to test than whether the global community, acting through the UN and the WHO, is really serious about its often stated aspiration to improve health for all and whether it is truly prepared to value every life equally. It is a test of our global institutions.

The relationship between private business and government goes beyond simply regulation if for no other reason than that Government is so often its biggest, if generally indirect, customer. Much of healthcare is subsidised by governments around the world. Even in the USA, where healthcare provision is largely private, the US Government pays approaching half the cost. Government can reasonably expect to have considerable influence over what commercial companies do.

The pharmaceutical industry is a very particular case that lives with a paradox. The public wants its products and it wants the new drugs that offer new hope of relief from pain and suffering, yet the pharmaceutical industry itself is amongst the least trusted and the most criticised, even reviled, in the world. The public want to believe in their drugs, yet there has been a history of half-truths, of concealed research findings and of hard selling. These practices may only apply to some parts of the industry but they have contaminated the image of the rest.

The heart of the problem lies in their business model. Pharmaceutical companies have to invest for many years in the development of a product, which may fail at any stage. They then have a limited period in which to sell the product before it comes out of patent. There are huge sunk costs and enormous risks before any drug comes to the market. Figure 8.4 illustrates the size of investment that has to be made over many years – the sunk costs – before the drug goes on sale and costs start to be recovered by income growth. Bad results in trials or when on public sale can lead to the drug being withdrawn at any stage and the sunk costs not being recovered.

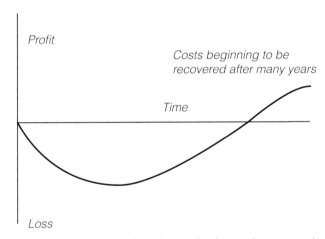

Figure 8.4 A pharmaceutical company's sunk costs that have to be recovered

This model will naturally induce certain behaviours. There is little wonder that some companies spend 40% of their turnover on sales and marketing and target individual doctors with gifts and skiing trips as well as product information. It is also likely to lead to a culture of secrecy, where the details of the development of a drug are kept out of the sight of competitors and the information given to the market is very carefully managed. At the best this secrecy is sensible commercial behaviour and at the worst it can lead to the concealing of important information, the failure to ask questions that might affect the future of the drug and ultimately to the harming of patients. It can certainly lead to mistrust.

There are various ways that governments have responded to these issues from legislating for more openness to, as in the UK, setting up its own process through the National

Institute for Health and Clinical Excellence (NICE) to assess new drugs and decide whether they should be made available on the NHS.

Initially there were many confrontations over the very existence of NICE, and it is still controversial. However, we are beginning to see agreements and compromises being struck between NICE and pharmaceutical companies over meeting the costs of certain drugs only where patients who are prescribed them actually benefit. It is a sort of 'payment by results' scheme. There are discussions about going further and having governments, or the big health systems such as the NHS, involved to some extent in the early research and development with some cost sharing and risk sharing.[28] There may perhaps even be learning to be had from the International Financing Facility for Immunization, which as we discussed earlier, subsidises the development of drugs needed in poor countries.

In the USA, as part of President Obama's reform plans, pharmaceutical companies and other suppliers are being asked to agree caps on future costs. Whilst these are not draconian, they do indicate that government, as a major indirect purchaser of drugs believes it has a role in cost control.

These are very big changes facing these enormous companies. However, they may only be the beginning. They face challenges from other biotech companies in their markets, whilst the pressure from people like Lee Hartwell to move to a more diagnostic-based early health model will affect their businesses. They will also be affected by the shifts of world power and the need to think about how to serve the 5 billion people who are likely over the next few years to enter the global marketplace in some form or other. All this will require new approaches and new business models.

Professor CK Prahalad, based at the Ross School of Business in Michigan, argues that we can already begin to see the new approaches that organisations will need to adopt to reach these people such as reducing costs, providing 'single serve' products and paying for usage, not ownership. He argues, in a concept that resonates with the theme of this book, that "when we start innovating at the bottom of the pyramid, many of the innovations will flow back to the developed world as well".[29]

Pharma, in common with other commercial organisations, will need to start to turn the world upside down. The ultimate test of course will be how much energy and effort they put into providing medicines for the bottom billion. This will be the test for their reputation, but also show whether they have understood the implications of the new global outlook and want to work with its flow. It is interesting to see that GlaxoSmithKline (GSK) is taking just such an initiative by offering to pool some patents and some research with competitors working in areas of interest to poor countries.

We are living through a financial and economic crisis which, whatever else its long-term impact, will change the relationship between financial and commercial interests and the state. It is very likely that the short-term role of the state in bailing out the bankrupt banks and shoring up commercial lending and other activity will be followed by some continuing state involvement.

Whilst the mid- and longer term consequences are unknown, it currently seems clear that the era of light touch regulation and of simply trusting the market to get it right is over. There are underlying trends that may make capitalism more, in Geoff Mulgan's words, "the servant and not the master of humanity".[30]

Health is probably slightly ahead of other sectors in this regard if for no other reason than because the unfettered private sector control of American healthcare has been seen to be a failure for so long. Other countries have been generally wary of copying what has been seen as a bursting bubble. Partly as a result, public–private partnerships of various kinds are amongst the richest areas of innovation in health. There is also a new vein of innovation coming from what is being called philanthro-capitalism, where foundations and individuals use their wealth to promote new enterprises and from organisations like the World Business Council for Sustainable Development, which believes that governments, businesses and international not-for-profit organisations cannot achieve sustainability on their own.

This mix of public and private, not-for-profit, cooperative and social enterprises will vary from country to country and offers enormous scope to expand and improve healthcare. In the end, however, in most rich societies at least, government has to take responsibility that goes beyond a purely regulatory function. Government, just as it did with the banks, has to stand behind the healthcare providers.

The fundamental point is that people have expectations of their government far wider than the purely commercial contract they may have with a healthcare provider. They expect government to be looking out for them, to ensure their health and, if regulation fails, step in. This is about a social contract, rather than a commercial one, and about government's responsibility to act for health as a public good and secure our right to health.

This was seen quite explicitly with the impending failure of the world's banking system. It will be seen equally clearly if governments fail to deal adequately with health crises in the future.

Conclusions

This and the previous chapter have been concerned with practical knowledge, by which I mean in very simple terms *what we need to know to get the right things done.*

In this chapter we have explored how the natural sciences and the new technologies are combining to create new and extraordinary opportunities to improve health in ways we could not have imagined 10 years ago. There is no reason to think that this progress will stop or even slow down over the next few years.

We have choices about how we use this new knowledge. We can use it to promote early health or keep the emphasis, as now, on tackling later disease. We can use it to promote independence or to strengthen dependence on the professional and the expert. We can use it to strive for equity or we can let it create further inequalities.

The last chapter also brought out the dependence the natural sciences have on the social sciences and on understanding of people, society, culture, economics and politics. All the purely scientific knowledge in the world won't help unless clinicians know how to apply it and, very often, how to persuade people to accept it. Moreover, patients themselves are central to health, they generally determine what happens as a result of any encounter with professionals and their engagement in every aspect of care is crucial. Developments in the natural and social sciences go hand in hand.

We have also seen in this chapter how health systems are so important in putting knowledge into practice and how methodologies are being developed to implement improvements and continuously improve quality. These methods bring with them a focus on the value of outcomes and shift away from the emphasis, which is so familiar in health care, on the continuing demand for more funding.

Finally, we have also seen how the boundaries are blurring between private business, government, social enterprises and not-for-profit activity as they enter into partnerships, alliances and joint ventures. Public opinion and the opportunities presented by these partnerships are steering the private sector ever more towards profitable ways to serve the public good.

Taken together these conclusions represent a very different picture from the simple model of western scientific medicine that we started with – with its belief in the power of science, its all powerful doctors, its use of the market to create improvement and its reliance on ever-increasing sums of both public and private money.

We will see in the next chapter how the paradigm is shifting.

References

1. Topol EJ. *Genomics of Cardiovascular Disease* in Opie LH, Yellon DM. *Cardiology at the limits X.* University of Cape Town Press. 2008.
2. Partnership for Personalized Medicine brochure. 2008.
3. Lee H. Cambridge University. Available at: www.haem.cam.ac.uk/ddu/.
4. Castell W. Speech at the Pacific Health Summit, Seattle, Washington 20–11 June, 2005.
5. Barker D. *Nutrition in the womb.* The Barker Foundation. 2008
6. International Financial Facility for Immunization. Available at: www.iff-immunisation.org/.
7. Taskforce on Innovative International Finance for Health Systems. *More Money for Health and More Health for Money.* 2009. Available at: www.internationalhealthpartnership.
8. Mundie C. Information technology; Advancing global health. *NBR Analysis* 2006; **17**: April.
9. Wooton M, Patil NG, Scott RE, Ho K. *Telehealth in the Developing World.* London: Royal Society of Medicine Press Ltd, 2009.
10. Boschi-Pinto C, Velevit L, Shibuya K. Estimating child mortality due to diarrhoea in developing countries. *Bull World Health Organ* [Online] 2008; **86**. Available at: www.scielosp.org/scielo.php?pid=S0042-96862008000900015&script=sci_arttext. [Accessed 20 September 2009].
11. United Nations Children's Fund. *State of the World's Children 2009: Maternal and newborn health 2009.* Available at: www.unicef.org/sowc09/docs/SOWC09-FullReport-EN.pdf.
12. VISION 2020. *The Right to Sight. Blindness and visual impairment: Global facts.* [Online]. Available at: www.v2020.org/page.asp?section=000100010036.
13. Pang T, Gray M, Evans T. The 15th Grand Challenge for global public health. *The Lancet* 2006; **367**: 284–6.
14. Gawande A, Berwick D, Fisher E, McClellan M. *10 Steps to better health care.* New York Times 13 August 2009.
15. Daar A, Singer P, Persaad D. Grand challenges in chronic non-communicable diseases. *Nature* 2007; **450**: 490–6.
16. Madon T, Hofman K, Kupfer L, Glass R. Implementation science. *Science* 2007; **318**: 1728–29.
17. Maximizing Synergies between Health Systems and Global Health Initiatives: Initial Summary Conclusions and Recommendations. Venice, July 2009.
18. Berwick D. In unpublished paper from Joe McCannon.
19. Institute for Healthcare Improvement. *About us* [Online]. Available at: www.ihi.org/ihi. [Accessed 20 September 2009].
20. Watcher RM, Pronovost PJ. The 100,000 Lives Campaign: A scientific and policy review. Journal on Quality and Patient Safety [Online] 2006; **32**: 621–7. Available at: psnet.ahrq.gov/public/Wachter_JCJQSH_2006.pdf.

21. McCannon CJ, Schall MW, Calkins DR, Nazem AG. *Saving 100 000 lives in US Hospitals.* BMJ. 2006; 332; 1328–1330.

22. Hackbarth A.D., McCannon C.J., Berwick D.M.: *Interpreting the "lives saved" result of IHI's 100,000 Lives Campaign.* Joint Commission Benchmark. 8:1–3, 10–11, Sept.–Oct. 2006.

23. NHS Modernisation Agency. *10 high impact changes for service delivery and improvement: a guide for NHS leaders.* NHS, UK 2004.

24. Institute of Medicine. *Crossing the quality chasm: a new health system for the 21st Century.* National academy Press, USA, 2001.

25. Rawlins M.D. *De Testimonio - On the evidence for decisions about the use of therapeutic interventions.* Harveian Oration. Royal College of Physicians, London. 2008.

26. World Econommic Forum: "*Forum funding to action: strengthening healthcare systems in Sub Saharan Africa*". June 2006.

27. World Health Organization. *Genomics and World Health.* Geneva 2002.

28. Cooksey D. *A Review of UK Health Research Funding.* TSO, London 2006.

29. Prahald C.H. *The fortune at the bottom of the pyramid: eliminating poverty through profits.* Wharton School Publishing. 2005.

30. Mulgan G. *After Capitalism.* Prospect. April 2009. 32–39.

9 The paradigm shift to global health

Hal Whitehead is a Professor of marine biology at the University of Dalhousie in Nova Scotia. He specialises in whales, which he studies from his sailing boat as, months at a time, he and they follow the winds and the currents through the oceans of the world.

Hal told me how he has several times talked with Inuit in the north of Canada about global warming and climate change. They reassured him that there was nothing to worry about. We were just in a period when the weather was warmer and the winds from a different direction. It would all change again, they told him. It always has.

He asked about the polar bears. He wondered if their habitat was threatened. The lack of ice in the summer meant they couldn't get near the seals on which they depended for meat and their numbers were already reducing. Nonsense, said the Inuit, there are more of them than ever. You see them all the time around the villages.

The Inuit were, of course, right. They saw more polar bears. With less ice, poorer hunting and a smaller area to roam, more polar bears had taken to visiting the villages and scavenging for what they could find around the human settlements.

Hal's experience with the Inuit reminded me of a passage in Tom Stoppard's play *Jumpers*. Meeting a friend in a corridor, Wittgenstein, the great Austrian philosopher, said: "Tell me, why do people always say it was natural for men to assume that the sun went round the earth rather than that the earth was rotating?" His friend said, "Well, obviously because it just looks as if the sun is going round the earth." To which the philosopher replied, 'Well, what would it have looked like if it had looked as if the earth was rotating?'

It certainly looked to the Inuit as if there were more polar bears.

A global perspective

It matters how we see the world because it determines how we act. People thought and acted differently when they believed that the sun went round the earth and that man was at the centre of the universe. When they began to change their perspective and see that the earth went round the sun it caused havoc with the established beliefs of the day. The Catholic Church and other authorities reacted with outrage and violence.

I don't want to overstretch the parallel, because there is more to it than this, but the change from seeing doctors at the centre of health – with the whole world of healthcare revolving around them – to recognising that it is actually the patient who is there, and who has been there all along (whatever it looked like to us at the time), will change the things we believe and the way we act.

Knowledge is useful but it only makes real sense when we put it in the context of how we see the world. Everything depends on our perspective and our view of the world. We need to re-visit the paradigm of western scientific medicine, which has for the last century dominated thinking about health and healthcare, and consider how it needs to change to fit into the environment and meet the needs of the twenty-first century.

There is a new set of values emerging that underlie these changes that reflect our interdependence, our desire for independence and the now widespread belief in a right to health.

Many people get this intuitively. They don't need to be told that the world is changing. Young people in particular, for whom this is the world they know, migrants and others have for years been talking about global health and values. Pioneers are putting these ideas into practice, academics are writing about them and policymakers are pronouncing. New technologies and the processes of globalisation add impetus to the changes. These things, taken together, make the process of change unstoppable.

I have described this book as a quest for understanding of what is happening in the world and a search for global health in the twenty-first century. We are approaching our goal and the task in this chapter is to put all the changes we have observed together in order to try to understand what between them they add up to and make explicit what is already implicitly understood by many.

The chapter starts with a discussion of the paradigm shift in western scientific medicine. It continues by investigating the underlying values and goes on to describe the movement of people and ideas that are making these changes real. We will look in the next chapter at what this means in practice and what we can do to accelerate and embed these changes.

Western scientific medicine

I said at the beginning of the book that western scientific medicine depended on the four features of greater professionalism, scientific discovery, commercial innovation and increased funding. We have discussed them all in the intervening chapters and shown how they are adapting to the new world.

I have used the idea of a paradigm in the book to mean a model and a way of thinking or – as I see from the Internet – *the set of values and concepts that represent an accepted way of doing things within an organisation or community.* This definition represents very well the way that these four features combine with others to create a particular and *accepted* way of looking at the world and acting.[2]

Similarly, the same source defines a paradigm shift as: *an adjustment in thinking that comes about as a result of new discoveries, inventions and real-world experiences.* This, too, describes well what is happening in the world of health and medicine. The twentieth-century paradigm is coming up against the discoveries, inventions and, above all, real-life experiences of the twenty-first century world.

Let us examine each of these four features of western scientific medicine in turn.

The changing nature of professionalism

A great deal of attention was given to increasing professional skills and improving professional standards throughout the last century. It has given us large numbers of highly capable doctors, nurses, midwives and other professionals who have conquered many conditions and contributed to our longevity and our health.

This process has also reinforced the power of these groups. Specialism and skills have given them knowledge and power over the layperson and given them an unrivalled position in negotiating with governments and authorities. Monopoly power has been accreted alongside the knowledge.

Andrew Cunningham and Bridie Andrews have argued that this has been a very long-term development and that by placing hospitals, clinics and professionals at the centre of healthcare and by focusing on diseases and physical processes, clinicians have come, consciously or unconsciously, to objectify and disempower patients.[3]

Whilst many thousands of professionals, through their own humanity and training, relate to their patients with the utmost sensitivity, the systems they work in reinforce their power and seem to disempower the patient at every turn. Despite this, as we discussed in Chapter 7, patients very often don't do as they are told or are advised, as the 30–50% of uncompleted courses of medication tell us.

In fact it is the other way up. Patients, rather than the professionals, more often decide what will actually happen. They subvert professional power. As we saw with the examples of lack of trust and the discussion of how social and cultural issues affect beliefs and behaviours, patients are very often in practice the people who empower and enable the professionals to act, rather than the other way round.

In reality patients are at the centre and have been all along. We have to change our perspective. There is a real shift in the paradigm here from the idea that professionals always know best to the idea that the professionals' competence is enhanced and enabled by the patients and communities they serve.

This is a transfer of power and as such is difficult and resented by some. In the hierarchical British NHS 20 years ago it was not uncommon to hear doctors complaining about patients' demands or about how they wanted to question or dispute the doctor's conclusions. Nowadays this is changing rapidly, driven partly by training, partly by generational change and partly by external factors such as politics, stronger management and the fact that, in some countries at least, patients sue.

These changes have provoked much debate about the future role of doctors and their relationship with other professionals, many of whom are increasingly well educated and taking over tasks that had previously only been done by doctors. I was at a meeting in Oxford where a panel of doctors and educators were discussing this and setting out their ideas. "What", the panel was asked, "was left that was unique to doctors alone?" It is quite a difficult question because it tempts people to mix emotion and dispassionate analysis, ideology and observable facts and can lead to some tendentious and muddled arguments.

Sir John Tooke, the Head of the Council of Deans of Medical Schools, gave a clear description of what medical schools aimed to equip doctors with: from the understanding of scientific principles to ethics and accountability. He said that members of any other profession could be as well equipped and knowledgeable in any of these areas as doctors, but that medical education was designed to ensure doctors were competent in every one of these areas. It was, although he didn't put it like this, a very objective description of what was special about doctors: the shared medical education.

One of the other panellists asked the audience to vote on whether each of us would rather see a doctor or a nurse if we were really ill. The big majority voted for a doctor, some of us abstained and nobody, as I recall, voted for a nurse. He felt he had made his point.

I on the other hand felt rather cheated. I know others did as well. The man next to me, the former Head of an Oxford College, leaned across and said that the speaker was just manipulating us with a gimmick. I had to leave the meeting early and it was as I was getting up to go, too late to make a protest that I realised what was wrong.

It was a question for the twentieth century.

We should never have allowed ourselves to be shoehorned with this simple and old-fashioned question. We should have asked "Which doctor? Which nurse?" before we were ready to reply. That would have been realistic twenty-first century behaviour. We were, after all, assertive patients and we wanted to understand our choices.

It is not just a question of whether a particular doctor or the nurse was competent, although that was also important. It was a question about their training, experience and skill. To take an obvious example, I am much more likely to benefit, as a middle-aged man, by being looked after by a specialist cardiac nurse rather than by an obstetrician. I have seen plenty of highly trained specialists, whether plastic surgeons or psychiatrists, defer to the nurse or other professional who understands another speciality better or has a particular skill.

The panellist was right that the average doctor has the broadest base of knowledge and skill and the deepest training, but that is a simple truism and misses the point that I want the right person for the job in hand. His question was redolent of all the twentieth-century assumptions about the relationships between doctors and patients and doctors and other professionals. These are, of course, assumptions shared by most patients and tend to shape our behaviour.

It reminded me of the very different attitude of Keith Willett, Professor of Trauma Surgery at the University of Oxford and National Clinical Director for Trauma. I remember him telling me when we worked together in Oxford that when you were in theatre or the Emergency room everybody had to leave his or her professional background outside the door. Inside everyone used the skills they had. Who did what depended on who was most skilled at doing it, not on their professional background.

It was this same attitude that had led Keith and colleagues to decide that only nurses could discharge patients from the trauma wards. The nurses spent more time with the patients and were better able to judge when they could go home. It was an attitude that turned traditional practice on its head and, for a time at least, greatly upset some of Keith's more traditional colleagues.

These simple stories describe something of the difficulties and tensions inherent in the changes underway. There are, however, more and more doctors like Keith who are turning the old view upside down.

Science in society

The ideas and approaches of western science have also dominated the world over the last few centuries and they, too, have delivered enormous benefits. There is undoubtedly much more to come.

In medicine the way that science is applied is absolutely key and policymakers talk about translational research and, more simply, how to transfer knowledge from the laboratory to the bedside or the home. Technological development, of course, plays a vital role in developing the devices and creating the applications that allow us to benefit from science. However, as we saw in the last chapter, the human and social aspects are also vitally important.

Knowledge of culture, society, psychology, politics and economics are central to successful application and the disciplines of operational research and implementation science rely on behavioural understanding and on experimentation in the real and untidy world. Some people argue that with the increase in non-communicable disease, linked as it is to behaviour, this interface between the social and natural sciences represents the most important areas for research today.

The IHI's quality improvement methodologies, described in the last chapter, use an understanding of how human beings and systems behave in helping people create local solutions, tailored to their own environment. Over more than 20 years, the IHI has demonstrated how quality improvement and the successful application of the discoveries of science depend both on re-designing systems and on understanding what happens in real life.

The ideas and approaches of western science are themselves conditioned by their social context. They represent one way of looking at the world and, in doing so, discount or ignore insights that may be available from other perspectives and other traditions of medicine. Chinese and African policymakers both now advocate the use of traditional medicine alongside western.

Dr Janet Smylie working in northern Canada has, as we saw earlier, argued that clinicians should look at and evaluate all the evidence, from traditional sources as well as from western science. This is a sophisticated approach that avoids the trap of saying it is either the one tradition or the other, but lays the stress on evaluation and evidence. A clinician who evaluates the evidence will throw out the nonsense and keep the sense from both traditions.

This discussion also brings out the point that clinicians need continually to evaluate the evidence even if they work exclusively within the western scientific tradition. In many cases there may not be very good evidence and clinicians may rely on a mixture of taking a logical and pragmatic approach and using their own experience.

The standard of knowledge and evidence we have may not be as conclusive and impressive as the public probably thinks it is. Even the results of the gold standard research – the double blind clinical trial – are limited in scope because they are based on the evidence from patients who do not have multiple conditions and complicating factors. As clinical friends have told me, and the literature attests, the task of diagnosis and treatment of an elderly patient with three or four conditions, for which they are taking a mix of medications, is no simple matter that you can look up in a textbook or on the Internet.

Clinicians evaluate the evidence. So too, as this book has asserted many times, do patients. Even when the clinician has settled on a course of action, the patient may need convincing or may simply make up his or her own mind and, intentionally or not, subvert the doctor's chosen route.

The final complication in using science in medicine, as we discussed in the last chapter, is that there are some fundamental choices about how to use the knowledge generated by science. It can be used to promote early health or keep the emphasis, as now, on tackling later disease. It can be used to promote independence or to strengthen dependence on the professional and the expert. It can be used to strive for equity or to create further inequalities.

We have seen in previous chapters how some of these choices are being made and how a great deal of research and development is being directed firmly towards dealing with specific problems. New business models have been created that fund research into the diseases of the poor, researchers are pursuing technological solutions to health problems and innovators are working to integrate scientific discovery directly into health systems. The UK, under the leadership of Dame Sally Davies, has taken a world lead in this with its research strategy entitled appropriately "Best Research for Best Health".

Medical science does not have to be fettered by the needs of today and the decisions of populations and policymakers. There is an important place and space for free and disinterested scientific discovery, but it is not the whole story. Science is made relevant by society and cultures; its application requires understanding people and society.

We have choices to make about the sorts of health systems we want and the sort of society we want to live in. We don't need to start, as western scientific medicine has traditionally done, by studying the science and then applying it to society but, rather, turn the world the other way up and start with understanding society and seek to apply the findings from both the natural and the social sciences.

This is a profound difference that influences the way that clinicians think and behave.

Commercial activity and public benefit

Scientific discovery and commercial interests have very often gone hand in hand in medicine. Commercial businesses have contributed enormously to research and the development of drugs, devices, services and facilities that have greatly benefited the public. Competition and the commercial drive for innovation have worked in the past and still work now. These enterprises have also, of course, reaped rich rewards, with health and healthcare now a significant segment of all stock markets and at least 16% of the world's largest economy dedicated to it.

Commerce has worked by identifying needs and gaps and creating products and by exploiting the products of scientific and technological research. It has focussed very largely in personal healthcare, selling products to be used by clinicians in looking after individuals rather than concentrating on population and public health. It has in healthcare, as elsewhere, followed the money.

The capacity to innovate comes at a price. Businesses that ally themselves with science and, particularly, with clinicians are in a very powerful position when it comes to marketing and sales. Patients and purchasers are often ill equipped to challenge them. Doctors advocating the purchase of particular drugs or treatments on television must be amongst the most powerful advertisers for any business in the world. Advertisements that say "Show your man you care, buy him a CT Scan for Christmas" are very compelling, regardless of the fact – not, of course, stated in the advert – that every unnecessary CT scan adds to the cancer risk.

Regulators and purchasers need to develop good systems to sort out the good from the bad and to make sure that they and patients are not purchasing snake oil, even if it is sometimes made from real snakes. The two systems of the USA and the UK have gone down different routes, with other countries adopting positions in between the two.

The US has relied on a licensing system run by the Food and Drug Administration (FDA) to ensure products are safe and then developed an extraordinarily bureaucratic insurance system that dictates what particular insurance companies will or won't pay for. This system has itself added an overhead of 15% to the total costs of the system and involved countless patients in long hours of negotiation. In addition individuals may choose to go outside the system and pay themselves for any therapy licensed by the FDA.

The UK has a parallel licensing authority, the Medicines and Healthcare products Regulatory Agency (MHRA), but has also introduced another check in NICE that compares therapies and, using both patient and scientific input, makes judgements about what therapies offer sufficient value to be worth using and paying for in the NHS. Patients may insure themselves separately as in the USA or go outside the system altogether and pay for any product licensed in the UK.

In principle the establishment of NICE was a fairly straightforward decision. Although it was established before I was appointed, as Chief Executive I wanted to know that the US$15 billion plus that we were spending on drugs was worthwhile and good value. It was really a 'no-brainer'. In practice, however, the operation of NICE has been very contentious, with pharmaceutical companies and some patient groups arguing that it has denied patients drugs that could benefit them. Others, however, have argued that it stopped money being spent on drugs, which might have been safe, but which had marginal if any benefits and then only in a few of the patients treated.

NICE is a true world leader that has generated interest in every country that is trying to control expenditure and counter commercial marketing. Over time as we saw in the last chapter, its operation and relationship with businesses has changed and new agreements are being reached where pharmaceutical companies agree to demonstrate specified levels of benefit to NHS patients from new drugs before NICE approves them for use in the NHS.

This is just one example of how commercial businesses and health are moving closer together, with the recognition of their interdependence. In the last chapter we saw how the boundaries are blurring between private business, government, social enterprises and not-for-profit activity as they enter into partnerships, alliances and joint ventures.

It appears that public opinion and the opportunities presented by these partnerships are steering the private sector ever more towards profitable ways to serve the public good. More generally there is a sense that capitalism is adapting to changed times in order to survive. Geoff Mulgan, the former head of the UK Government Strategy Unit, has argued that the credit crunch and financial crisis has changed things materially with the death of the simple notion that free markets can provide what the world needs and that we are all able to act as rational economic beings. He believes that we are entering a new era where markets and capitalism will serve humanity, rather than the other way round.[4]

The world it appears is turning upside down. Commerce and capitalism have recognised, for the next few years at least, that the greatest financial gains in healthcare are to be had in working with others for the public good and not just for the benefits of private individuals. Private investment will be at its most effective by working with others to achieve wider goals.

Funding and value

The other main feature of western scientific medicine has been the relentless demand for more expenditure throughout the last 100 years – with the apparent supposition that more is always better, despite much evidence to the contrary. This feature is as ingrained into the psyche of health workers as any of the others and is as difficult to influence.

Francis Omaswa from Uganda gives the lie to this when he talks of poor countries not being able to afford waste. When money is short every penny counts. It is only in richer countries that we can afford to be profligate, throwing money at problems and failing to search out value. There are undoubtedly places where more money is needed, including health services in Uganda, but even there new money needs to be spent well to achieve the desired outcomes.

Many attempts have been made to try to define productivity in healthcare although with little success. Many of the formulas used are borrowed from industrial production models and are misleading and simplistic. At their worst they can make policymakers focus on units of activity and not outcomes as being the end goal of healthcare.

Two simple examples from the UK illustrate different aspects of the problem. One example is that a hospital may be paid each time a patient, let us say an elderly woman, is admitted to hospital during a cold winter, but receive little or nothing if a smart clinician works out how to keep her fit and healthy at home. If we think in terms of simple productivity, then the more admissions the better. If we think in terms of health outcomes, home is almost certainly best. The incentives are wrong.

Health is not alone in having these difficulties. Until recently, fire service productivity in the UK was measured in terms of the number of fires dealt with. Here, too, the more fires the better! Cure was incentivised over prevention.

On the other hand, it is important to make sure that facilities are well utilised and these sort of production models are useful in considering utilisation rates and down time in operating theatres and, no doubt, in fire stations.

These examples show how difficult it is to produce figures that can give a sense of the overall productivity of a health system. Various complex formulations have been created. In the NHS for example, we attempted to give cash values to benefits such as improved health or reduced waiting times and measure changes in productivity by relating these to the cost of producing them. The figures were as good as the assumptions we made.

A better approach is surely that adopted by the IHI and others who, in developing methods to implement improvements and improve quality, treat cost as another variable input to be managed. These methods bring with them a focus on the value of outcomes and shift away from the emphasis on inputs, which is so familiar in health care. This new approach, named Triple Aim, integrates cost management into population health and individual healthcare. These methods allow for the benchmarking of cost and outcomes, offering a measure of comparative value.

This is the area where the paradigm shift that we are discussing has furthest to go. The issue is complicated by the fact that more money is undoubtedly needed in many countries. A billion people still receive no healthcare at all, however even there the focus needs to be on how any money that is available is used. Globally, the direction of travel is clear, but much more needs to be done to ensure that measures of input spending are replaced by credible measures of the social and economic value achieved.

Taken together, the changes described here add up to a shift in the paradigm of western scientific medicine and the creation of a new way of looking at the world in terms of global health. This shift is summarised in Figure 9.1.

- *Greater professional competence is achieved through patients and communities empowering and working with professionals*
- *Scientific discovery is made relevant by our understanding of society and of how to apply it*
- *Commercial innovation is most effective in working with others to achieve wider goals*
- *Measures of input spending are replaced by measures of the social and economic value achieved*

Figure 9.1 The paradigm shift towards global health

The values of global health

This way of looking at the world is no more neutral or value free than any other. There are other perspectives that may be based on very different values, drawn from religion, culture or tradition. As we saw with the Inuit and Professor Whitehead, different perspectives will lead people to believe very different things and take very different actions.

I have described this book as a search for global health. It is an attempt to understand a movement of people and ideas that is gathering momentum. It is gradually shifting the way we think about health and healthcare and altering the paradigm or model we carry in our heads.

We no longer believe, to parody only a little, that the doctor is always right, science will give us all the answers, we can leave everything to the market and that more expenditure means better health. We see all these things differently now. This changed perspective is accompanied by a new set of values, by which I mean beliefs about what we think is important and that influence the way we behave. The discussion in this book suggests that the values associated with the idea of global health fall into three groups.

The first group is essentially about valuing everything to do with our interdependence including the belief that we are all of equal value, that our interconnections and interactions add value, that we all have something to teach and something to learn, that what affects one affects us all and that we will benefit from sharing and mutual respect.

The second area concerns our independence and what I have described, following Amartya Sen, as being the independence to live a life we have reason to value. It is about valuing our individual identity and our personal beliefs, culture, tradition and autonomy.

The third area, which in some ways reconciles the potential tension between our independence and our interdependence, is about human rights in general and the right to health in particular. It encompasses beliefs in the value of fairness, accountability and transparency.

These three groups – interdependence, independence and rights – are in many ways universal. They are features of globalisation and apply to areas other than health. We will discuss their implications briefly in turn.

Interdependence and the need to act accordingly

The theme of interdependence has run throughout this book and is manifest in many ways from our shared vulnerability to pandemics to our reliance on the same pool of health workers and the same scientific research. The implications of this have not yet been fully understood. There is still, for example, a division in our thinking between what happens in health in poor countries and in rich. Apart from where there is obvious overlap, such as with pandemics, we still tend to think about them and treat them separately.

In particular we do not, as in the theme of this book, generally try to transfer knowledge from poorer to richer countries but only see knowledge transfer as going the other way. We also tend to neglect the fact that when rich and poor countries work together on a problem they both gain. We in the UK can learn about TB from working with colleagues in Africa, where they have more experience of the disease. Our young people can learn from working for a period in Pakistan just as Pakistanis can learn from the UK. Benefits are mutual. There are opportunities for shared learning and co-development.

This has already been very simply demonstrated by the stories throughout this book of people from the UK working in Africa or Asia and learning as well as contributing. It has also been shown by the critical necessity of countries working together to deal with the shared risks of pandemics and the potential and dangers of exploitation of developments in genetics.

Health, in this context, sits within a wider framework of global cooperation, where we need to find ways of sharing the burden of climate change and dealing with the economic crisis and the other impending crises such as overpopulation. The United Nations (UN), through the WHO and other bodies, provides the forum and framework for creating the collective will and policy to tackle health issues and promote wider development.

This approach is still, as I argued in Chapter 5, relatively top down with the richer countries and global organisations doing international development, as it were, to the others. There is not, as yet, a clear or strong notion of co-development, an approach whereby we recognise that we are working together on the same issues and do so with mutual respect and understanding.

The Commission on Africa went some way towards this by saying: "What we are suggesting is a new kind of development, based on mutual respect and solidarity, and rooted in a sound analysis of what actually works". It went on to talk about what in Zulu and other Bantu languages is called *ubuntu*, which insists that "the very identity of each person is bound up with others in a community of all. I am what I am because of who we all are".[5]

There is a need to develop these ideas further and to move beyond the split of countries between developed and developing; we all have development needs, some are shared and some are local. We need to tackle the shared issues together and to learn from each other about how to tackle the local ones. The practical task is to find ways of making this happen in reality.

Independence

Health, science and technology have emancipated many people in richer countries from the day-to-day burdens of life and freed them to develop their own individuality and follow their own ideas and dreams wherever they may take them. At the same time the global movement of people has led to a far greater diversity of people, with different beliefs and habits, living in the same area.

These now well-established trends have enormous implications for health with the need to make services and health workers much more attuned and sensitive to this diversity of individuals and of peoples. This is already beginning to happen in many areas and clinicians in some areas of cities like London, New York, Toronto and Paris see the world in all its variety of background and lifestyle walk through their surgery doors.

In addition the value given to our personal independence means that health services and health policy need to become far closer than they are today to other areas such as education, employment and social support. As we saw in the early chapters, which dealt with health and poverty and health and wealth, our health is inextricably linked to social factors and social structures. Moreover, our ability to function independently depends on education as much as it does on health and our economic status.

Health as a human right and a public good

The belief that there is a right to health also has profound implications. The idea itself is not new, but it has been a long time in being put into practice in anything like a universal or consistent fashion.

The 1948 General Assembly of the United Nations set out that "Everyone has the right to a standard of living adequate for the health and well-being of himself and his family, including . . . medical care and the necessary social services".[6]

Since that rather qualified assertion of a right to health, there have been many others that have gradually deepened and clarified the idea, such as the European Union pronouncement in 2000 that "Everyone has the right of access to preventive health care and the right to benefit from medical treatment under the conditions established by national laws and practices"[7] and the African Union's *Africa Health Strategy 2007 to 2015*, which takes health being a human right as one of its central priniciples.

Over the last 60 years the notion that health is a human right has gradually become accepted in much of the world. Whilst there is much more to do to win the argument everywhere, attention has shifted to asking what this really means in practice in an area where there is massive scope for misunderstanding and confusion.

President Mary Robinson is determined to make assertions of human rights into practical propositions. She set up Realizing Rights in 2002 in order "to put human rights standards at the heart of global governance and policy-making and to ensure that the needs of the poorest and most vulnerable are addressed on the global stage."[8]

President Robinson was the first woman to be President of Ireland and is a former United Nations High Commissioner for Human Rights. She has that quiet authority that some leaders have where they are able to combine great passion and commitment with the humility to listen to other points of view. She is a consensus builder and healer as well as a visionary leader.

Her approach to rights, which she describes as "ethical globalisation", takes the simple assertion of rights a step further by providing a practical framework for action that eloquently reflects the values of global health. It:

- acknowledges shared responsibilities for addressing global challenges and affirms that our common humanity doesn't stop at national borders.
- recognises that all individuals are equal in dignity and have the right to certain entitlements, rather than viewing them as objects of benevolence or charity.
- embraces the importance of gender and the need for attention to the often different impacts of economic and social policies on women and men.
- affirms that a world connected by technology and trade must also be connected by shared values, norms of behaviour and systems of accountability.[9]

Paul Hunt as the UN Special Rapporteur on the right to health has taken the definition of health as a human right further by pointing out that this is not, for example, about the right of an individual woman to have the gynaecologist of her choice but the right of a population to have access to healthcare.[10]

These refinements begin to make the grand proclamation of the 1948 UN General Assembly practical and achievable by moving the debate away from impossibly impractical-sounding notions of individual rights and individualism to the rights we share and our right to partake in shared resource, shared entitlement and shared progress. It bridges our independence and our interdependence.

The right to health finds expression in Britain's NHS and other European and European-style health systems that have at their heart the idea that the health of all citizens is important to us all – that in economists' terms, health is a public good – and that health services should be available to all. The UK has been explicit both in the original 1946 Act establishing the National Health Service that healthcare should be available to all equally and more recently in the NHS Constitution asserting that the NHS belongs to the people.[11,12]

The right to health and the associated idea that, at least, basic health services should be available to everyone without user charges have gathered momentum in recent years and are now the focus of coordinated lobbying globally to implement this in the poorer countries of the world. This perspective sees the provision of healthcare to the poor as no longer being about aid and service but being about rights and entitlement. As the Commission for Africa says: "It is a journey from charity to justice".[5]

Meanwhile the great powers, old and new, of the USA and China are this year finding their own ways to extend healthcare coverage amongst their populations. President Obama is engaged in a very public and difficult battle in the USA to extend insurance cover to all US citizens, whilst China announced in May that it was developing a new health service for its population.

With these developments gathering momentum, Dr Gorik Ooms has more radically called for the development of a global social protection scheme. He notes that some countries will not in the foreseeable future be able to fund a health system for their people and will continue to be dependent on aid. Why not, he argues, make a permanent transfer of funds from richer countries to the poorest ones that would allow them to provide some social protection for their population? Why not see this as a small part of the richer countries' own health budgets? This would in effect mean that a country had a health budget, most of which was spent on its own people, but a small part of which was paid into a global fund in recognition that we are all interdependent globally. It is an inspiring idea. Supported by the Hélène De Beir Foundation, he is developing the idea further.

Linked to rights, but separate from them, is the demand for greater openness and accountability at every level of authority from the individual clinician to the pharmaceutical company, the government or intergovernmental organisation and the media.

The universal demand is for transparency and accountability with civil society groups that focus on this growing fast around the world. Whilst the roots of this activity go back decades and perhaps centuries, there is a pronounced shift now taking place towards a different sort of politics, which takes place outside formal institutions, and the creation of a more networked and engaged democracy.

Democracy has sometimes received a bad press down the centuries. Plato describes it scathingly as the system where every man's opinion is treated as being equally valid, whatever it is really worth.[14] Churchill said that it was the worst system apart from all the others.[15] More recently, I have heard civil servants speak of their minister's temper tantrums or other bad personal behaviour as "the price we have to pay for democracy".

Perhaps we should be thinking about this rather differently. One person, one vote is the foundation of democracy. In practice one of its main characteristics is fast becoming the idea that anyone and everyone can ask for information or expect an explanation of actions or policy.

The British civil service is non-political and has traditionally seen part of its role as speaking truth unto power. Updating this for the twenty-first century, we can see the

---

Interdependence – *living and interacting in an interconnected world with mutual respect and to mutual benefit*

Independence – *and the ability to live a life we have reason to value*

Rights – *the right to health backed up by transparency and accountability*

Figure 9.2 Three groups of values underpinning the new paradigm of global health

civil society movements are beginning to create mechanisms for making sure that power speaks truth unto us.

These three groups of values are very closely linked and can be described simply in Figure 9.2.

A movement of people and ideas

Whilst I have laboured in these pages to try to understand what is happening in health and searched for what global health might really mean, many young health professionals understand it intuitively.

There is a general truth that many young people in rich countries brought up on information and communication technology (ICT) and able from an early age to interact virtually with their peers of practically every race and creed, even if only through war games or shared tastes in music, have an awareness of the world and see international boundaries quite differently from their parents.

Every generation has different characteristics. Some commentators today believe that the generation coming of age around the turn of the century in rich countries are searching for meaning in their lives. They want to make a difference. Many have been brought up in some comfort, but are very aware of all the problems facing the world. They want to do things that make their actions and lives worthwhile and meaningful.

Some of this is perhaps reflected in their interest in international development and the campaigns to end poverty and raise awareness and funds for charitable causes. There has been a surge of interest in doing some development work, perhaps teaching in a school or working on an environmental project, during the 'gap' year between school and university.

Against this general background of idealism and interest in global issues, young health professionals, particularly doctors, have been developing their own approaches. I have met young people in the UK and USA who are interested in the health issues that affect the whole world, whether it is the environment, the migration of health workers, poverty or the status of women and want to explore its effect on health. They respect the science of their chosen discipline of medicine but want to understand how it applies to the world as it is with all its political, social, economic and environmental complexity. They are interested in global health.

This is not totally new. The International Federation of Medical Student Associations (IFMSA) was formed in 1951 and currently has as its mission "to offer future physicians a comprehensive introduction to global health issues".[16] Interest in global health has, however, really taken off in a big way the last few years with organisations and individuals developing ideas and acting on them.

Here I will touch briefly on the situation in the UK, which I know best. In doing so I recognise that the changes I describe here have been moving at a similar or faster pace in the USA and elsewhere. There are two main organisations in the UK: Medsin for medical students and Alma Mata for young doctors. Both now welcome people from any discipline into membership. Leaders of the two organisations have told me that they believe that around half of all medical students were interested in global health. This is reflected in the fact that about 40% of students out of a possible 8000 chose to go to developing countries as part of their 'elective' study period in 2004.[17] Some go for much longer periods.

They also told me that a much smaller number would be likely to pursue this interest in any practical fashion on into their later careers as the need for income and advancement took hold. Nevertheless, they made the point that the things they needed to think about as part of global health, such as poverty, disadvantage and exclusion, also applied to people in the UK, citing the example of unemployed workers and run down towns. Thinking in terms of global health is relevant in rich countries as well as poor. We need clinicians who understand global health in London as well as in Lusaka.

Theirs is a very modern outlook on the world, saying in a proposal on medical education that:

> "Global health is a field of practice, research and education focussed on health and the social, economic, political and cultural forces that shape it across the world. The discipline has a historical association with the distinct needs of developing countries but it is also concerned with health-related issues that transcend national boundaries and the differential effects of globalisation. It is a cross-disciplinary field, blending perspectives from the natural and social sciences and the humanities to understand the social relationships, biological processes and technologies that contribute to the improvement of health worldwide".[18]

There are risks in adopting this global outlook. Stoppard's Wittgenstein example referred directly to Galileo's experience. He attempted to demonstrate to the church and state authorities in seventeenth-century Italy that the earth went round the sun. They weren't having any of it and invoked the very word of God to prove that he was wrong. Galileo was disgraced and the Catholic Church and the State were stranded in the past by their own beliefs.

Anyone attempting to turn the world upside down today may face similar opposition. There will not be threats of execution or jail, but there may well be excommunication from the job market. There is no evidence, as yet, that the clinics and hospitals of the rich countries are looking for global health specialists or even generalists. In general, the opposite is true, with young doctors expected to keep to a very prescribed career path if they want to progress and succeed. Too strong an interest in global health may damage your immediate job prospects.

Medsin and Alma Ata are pressing to change this and to ensure that global health is included in the medical curriculum and that UK career structures can be adapted to allow people to work and train in poor countries for periods without losing out on their training accreditation and job prospects. They point out that a period in a poor country where disease may be more prevalent and resources far less can offer them much faster learning than in the controlled conditions of the UK.

Trainees will understand in a poor environment, far better than in the UK, why public health and primary care are so important and see at first hand the results of failure to treat early and prevent accidents and disease. Harking back to the experience of the consultant anaesthetist in southern Ethiopia that I described earlier, they will also have to learn to improve their clinical skills of listening to and observing the patient in the absence of all the machinery they have the use of in UK hospitals.

There is real sympathy and empathy for the young people interested in global health amongst their seniors. In the USA I heard Professor Mike Merson of Duke's Global

Health School refer to global health as being like Vietnam for many in his generation of Americans – something into which many young people poured their idealism. In the UK I heard Professor Sir John Tooke of the Peninsular Medical School say that he thought young people today were as idealistic about global health as our generation had been about the NHS.

The University authorities and Deans of the medical schools in the USA are listening to the young and setting about creating new global health courses. In an impressive example of how well American market forces can work, I recall attending a meeting at the University of California in San Francisco where deans from leading universities across the USA debated the content and curricula of global health masters and doctorates and discussed how they would be taught, examined and accredited.

They were responding to the demands of their customers, the young clinicians and scientists and trying to work out exactly what this notion of global health meant in practice. Meanwhile, back in the less market-driven UK, Sir John Tooke and his colleagues have set about finding ways to enable their students to follow up their interest in global health and even to have part of their training in poor countries.

Migrant health workers

Another group of people also understand these issues well. One of the results of the large-scale migration of health workers is that there are now many thousands of people with a view of the world from at least two different national perspectives and, often, from several more. Many of them are professionally trained and they have moved to places where the science was the same, but where they needed to learn to adapt their behaviours and adopt new practices.

The picture here is much more complicated than it is with the young professionals. It is impossible to generalise about the attitudes of such a diverse group of people coming, as they do, from very different backgrounds and having left their home countries under very different circumstances.

Governments and development agencies are now asking seriously what contribution these diasporas of people can make to health in both their original and adopted countries. Can their national and cultural ties and their more global outlook be used to help improve health?

In some ways the role that the diaspora can play in improving health in the countries of their families' origin is the most obvious part. The British Nigerian Dr Titilola Banjoko is the forceful and energetic Director of Africa Recruit, which works to find ways that expatriate Africans can contribute in all sectors through volunteering, returning home or providing investment in Africa.[19] She finds herself more and more in demand to give advice and offer ideas to governments and development agencies about how they can work with the different groups.

There are plenty of ideas and many good examples of, for instance, Ghanaian doctors returning home to work for periods in the Ghanaian Health Service. However the activities are not yet organised at any scale, the practical difficulties and barriers have not yet been overcome and there is not even enough information about the people who make up the diasporas and their skills, interests and attitudes.

There are also serious risks. Will health workers returning from the UK and the USA just import some of the unhelpful habits of the rich countries, which we have talked about so much in this book? How will the African British and the African American behave and be received? Will they be accepted or shunned by the people who stayed at home? Have they the right skills and attitudes to contribute?

Over time, however, as people like Lola Banjoko work at it, there is enormous scope here to share and learn and make a big impact on the health of people in poor countries.

There is also, although this goes beyond the scope of this book, a great opportunity to enhance the contribution migrants make to the receiving country. They may often be treated poorly, as we saw in Chapter 4. In reality they can offer different perspectives and skills.

The academics and policymakers

Governments and policy and policymakers are catching up. The UK Government published its first comprehensive policy statement *Health is Global* in 2008.[20] It identifies areas where the UK can add value to international efforts through building on its strengths, such as disease surveillance and education, as well as addressing the risks that threaten the health of the UK population. In 2009 the American Institute of Medicine delivered a report to the public and private sectors recommending action.[21] There is now also a rich and growing academic literature that is starting to describe and define the central elements of global health and provide the intellectual underpinning for the new discipline.

The academics and policymakers add weight and help generate momentum for the move towards global health. Continuing momentum is provided by the literally thousands of health workers and academics who are now communicating with each other and working together electronically.

We can of course now communicate so much better and quicker than ever before. Health professionals and researchers have been quick to take advantage of it. So too has the general public. I recall being told that whereas pornography was originally the most searched for topic on the Internet, health has now overtaken it with millions of people looking up symptoms, discussing their ideas and learning about diseases, treatments and developments.

An important feature of this increase in communication has been the growth of social networking and the development of 'communities of practice' amongst health professionals. They use these communities to spread ideas, to question and discuss and to create bonds and a sense of community amongst widely dispersed people.

Doctors.net.uk is a fascinating modern phenomenon. The brainchild of Dr Neil Bacon, he created it as a young doctor in Oxford because he saw the need for some way of connecting up doctors so that they could talk to each other virtually, exchanging information, accessing knowledge and building a network. His simple vision was of building a community, creating a virtual doctors mess where doctors could meet and discuss things in private, asking for advice, swapping ideas or just gossiping as they did in the real mess. It is run by doctors for doctors.

It is based on an equally simple business model. All doctors registered with the UK's General Medical Council can join free, but no one else can. They get an email address, A.Doctor@doctors.org.uk, free emails and access to any of the website's discussion forums, bulletin boards and other services. They can, for example, join a forum for trainee renal physicians and discuss issues of current concern and at the same time join in debate about current NHS policy or employment issues.

They can also post a question about their diagnosis or treatment of a patient on a bulletin board. Within a few hours they will receive comments or advice from other doctors, all of whom are identified by name, grade and employer. They are able to consult professional colleagues in real-time online.

In return for these services, Doctors.net.uk uses its unique membership to sell market research to people who may want to know what doctors think about a clinical or a political issue and to make evidence about new treatments and drugs available to doctors in membership. The NHS also uses it to deliver training and awareness packages; successfully, for example, raising awareness amongst doctors about how to contain methicillin-resistant *Staphylococcus aureus* (MRSA).

The deal is simple. Doctors.net.uk makes sure that any material and training or awareness programmes meet its standards for proof and objectivity. It promotes the scientific results of trials of drugs, for example, not straight advertising. In return doctors are willing to participate in surveys and training and, often welcome the promotional material about new treatments and drugs relevant to their speciality or interests.

Doctors.net.uk has today, in 2009, about 155 000 members, more than 90% of the total in the UK. It is used by 35 000 people every day.[22] It is now a real, if unacknowledged, part of the UK's health system and something of a model for what could be done elsewhere.

There is enormous potential to use this sort of technology to share knowledge and to support isolated clinicians anywhere in the world. Doctors.net.uk already has its stories from the developing world with, for example, a British doctor in Sri Lanka accessing it shortly after the Asian Tsunami in 2006 to seek advice about how to make potentially contaminated water drinkable.

Network 2015, a professional network for paediatricians, has a better story in which a British doctor in the Sudan wanted, and received, advice on whether a newborn child whose mother was dead could safely drink camel's milk. He could. The humble mobile phone network can currently top them all, however, with the account of how in late 2008 a doctor in England briefed a doctor in Africa on how to amputate a shoulder, taking him step by step through the process, live, as it happened, by text message.

In a few years' time these examples will undoubtedly seem commonplace and not worth writing about. As I write, however, they are still remarkable and dependent on the work of pioneering groups and individuals. We are perhaps nearing the point where policymakers embrace them as a central part of their thinking, but we are not there yet. Too often I have heard people dismiss these developments as too high tech for poor countries and been told that Broadband is too slow in Africa and electricity supplies too intermittent. These are both true, but pioneers, being pioneers, are finding ways round this.

Lord and Lady Roger and Jean Swinfen have used the Swinfen Trust to link volunteer clinicians in rich countries with clinicians working in 45 of the poorer countries of the world, ranging from Malawi and Cote d'Ivoire to Afghanistan and Uzbekistan. They have deliberately used the simplest technology available, email.

A clinician in Mali can write an email request for advice on a particular patient or condition and receives an answer from a clinician in Scotland. This being a global initiative, the Swinfens, based in the UK, have used the Australian University of Queensland as the terminus where the emails are received and sent on to the consulting clinicians. It works. More than 1700 requests were handled in 2008[23] up from 400 in 2000.

The University of Iowa Public Health Department, under the leadership of Professor Thomas Cook, has used a proprietary product, the eGranary, to store material downloaded from the Internet at times when there is electricity and Internet access. Clinicians and teachers locally can extract materials from the memory of the eGranary as and when they need it and power is available.[24]

These few examples, which represent only a very small part of the schemes that exist, show that there are ways round today's limitations that allow something of the potential of these communication and computing technologies to be realised. These innovative approaches are capable of removing distance and bringing knowledge and expertise to the remotest and loneliest parts of the globe. They build on and draw strength from the natural community and solidarity that most clinicians, wherever they are, feel for each other.

A community of course can exclude as well as include. Not everyone shares the sort of global outlook that I am describing here. Not everyone wants to share in it, of course, and some political regimes actively discourage their people from participating in the global community in this way. Others use these sorts of networks for their own purposes, good or evil. The technology is only a tool.

The outlook – risks and opportunities

This chapter has been an exploration of a developing global outlook in health in the twenty-first century. This way of looking at the world encompasses a sense of interdependency and mutuality, a breaking down of barriers of all sorts between sectors and societies and a strong framework of values about independence, rights, transparency and accountability. It is an optimistic viewpoint.

It is not yet fully coherent or fully realised, as our exploration in this chapter has shown. We need to understand what rights mean in practice, we need new models for public–private partnerships and for holding authorities to account. We don't yet know how the rise of China and India will affect it. These, however, are the questions we will want answered in the next few years. This is very much a developing outlook.

This chapter has, however, shown how far we have travelled from the ideas that made us so successful in the twentieth century. We share a respect for the natural sciences and for learning and professionalism but we no longer have the same insularity of approach, the same ideas about race and society, the same belief in the value of multinational corporations and American business method and the same respect for hierarchies. These were the attitudes that shaped policy and influenced behaviour for much of the last century.

The developing outlook is important because it is already influencing policy and behaviour amongst health workers and it will shape much of what happens for at least the early part of this century.

There are risks, however. It is an outlook shared by many health workers around the world, but primarily by those who have the money and the time to travel and to interact, virtually or in reality, with others from outside their immediate community. It is by its nature both value driven and elitist. It leaves some people out and it alienates others.

Whilst it is optimistic, it need not be naïve. There is an enormous amount to do to spread these ideas further and to gain the benefits they can bring. The old model of the twentieth century will not give way easily and vested interests will want it to continue. We need to understand how best to overcome these obstacles and add further momentum to this movement of people and ideas. This is the subject of the next chapter.

References

1. Stoppard T. *Jumpers*. Avalon. 1972.
2. Rudolph P, Pendill J. *Mosby's Dental Dictionary*. 2nd edition. St Louis: Elsevier, 2004.
3. Cunningham A, Andrews B. *Western Medicine as Contested Knowledge: Studies of imperialism*. Manchester: Manchester University Press, 1997.
4. Mulgan G. *After Capitalism*. Prospect. April 2009. 32–38.
5. Commission for Africa. *Our common interest*. [Online]. 2005. Available at: www.commissionforafrica.org/english/report/introduction.html.
6. United Nations. Article 25, *The Universal Declaration for Human Rights*. 1948. [Online]. Available at: www.un.org/en/documents/udhr/. [Accessed 23 September 2009].
7. European Commission. Article 35, *Charter of Fundamental Rights*. 2005. Available at: ec.europa.eu/justice_home/unit/charte/en/charter-solidarity.html. [Accessed 24 September 2009].
8. *Realising Rights: the ethical globalisation initiative* [Online]. Available from: www.realizingrights.org/index.php?option=com_content&task=view&id=46&Itemid=88. [Accessed 24 September 2009].
9. *Realising Rights: the ethical globalisation initiative. What is ethical globalisation?* [Online]. Available at: www.realizingrights.org/index.php?option=com_content&task=view&id=66&Itemid=109. [Accessed 24 September 2009].
10. Office of the United Nations High Commissioner for Human Rights. *The right to health*. [Online]. Fact sheet No. 31. Available at: www.ohchr.org/Documents/Publications/Factsheet31.pdf.
11. National Health Service Act 1946.
12. NHS for England. *NHS Constitution: The NHS belongs to us all* [Online] 21 January 2009. Available at: www.dh.gov.uk/prod_consum_dh/groups/dh_digitalassets/documents/digitalasset/dh_093442.pdf.
13. Ooms G. *The right to health and the sustainabiity of health care: why a new global health aid paradigm is needed*. 2008.
14. Plato. *The Republic*. 360 BC.
15. Gilbert M. *The Will of the People: Churchill and parliamentary democracy*. Toronto: Vintage Canada, 2006.
16. International Federation of Medical Students' Associations. Available at: www.ifmsa.org/. [Accessed 24 September 2009].
17. Miranda JJ, Yudkin JS, Willcott C. International health electives: four years of experience. *Travel Medicine and Infectious Diseases* 2005; **3**: 133–41.
18. Alma Mata. *Alma Mata Proposal for Postgraduate Training on Global Health, March 2009* [Online]. Available at: www.almamata.net/news/system/files/Postgraduate%20training%20in%20Global%20Health%20Proposal.pdf. [Accessed 24 September 2009].
19. Africa Recruit. Available at: www.africarecruit.com/.
20. Donaldson L. *Health is Global: proposals for a UK Government wide strategy*. [Online]. Available at: www.dh.gov.uk/en/Publicationsandstatistics/Publications/PublicationsPolicyAndGuidance/DH_072697.
21. Committee of the US Commitment to Global Health. *The U.S. Commitment to Global Health: Recommendations to the public and private sectors*. Institute of Medicine. May 2009. Available at: www.iom.edu/?ID=67183.

22. Doctors.net.uk. Available at: www.doctors.net.uk/.
23. Swinfen Charitable Trust. *Achievements* [Online]. Available at: www.swinfencharitabletrust.org/index. php?option=com_content&view=article&id=46&Itemid=55. [Accessed 24 September 2009].
24. The eGranary digital library. Available from: www.widernet.org/digitallibrary/. [Accessed 24 September 2009].

10 Action

I was sitting in the autumn sunshine on the Terrace of the House of Lords in London, overlooking the Thames and listening to a group of young people from Africa, the USA and the UK telling me about what they were doing in Sierra Leone. Here at this former heart of empire, black and white, male and female, a mix of professions and backgrounds, we talked together about what could be done.

They had arrived 3 years before as volunteers at the only children's hospital in Sierra Leone and were shocked by what they found.

The country was recovering from civil war and the Freetown hospital reflected it in every way: damaged, neglected and dirty. Mothers and fathers, like lost and bewildered refugees, were carrying their children as they wandered through its wards in search of help. The young people found a dead baby on a windowsill but no doctors anywhere. They discovered the next day that they all, the few there were, had been away on a training course.

Three years later, the young people are still there, having founded a charity, *Welbodi*, to support their work. Slowly and painstakingly they are assisting in the resurrection of the hospital, helping to instil some order into the chaos they found and providing services for a very needy population.

On the other side of the continent, and at about the same time the young people had arrived in Freetown, Dr Stephen Malinga had just become the Health Minister for Uganda. Tall, dark and heavily bearded he had been an obstetrician and gynaecologist in Chicago for several years. He had only returned to Uganda when his father died, in order to take over as head of the family. I have heard other Africans refer to him approvingly as a 'good African' for taking his family responsibilities seriously enough to come home and for maintaining his family farm and cows.

I met him again 3 months later, after he had done a comprehensive tour of health facilities in the country. He was in shock. It was so much worse than even he had expected. The facilities, the staffing levels and the quality of the service had all shocked him. As we talked he was still casting around for ideas, wondering where best to start and how he could have the greatest impact. He now fully understood what he had taken on.

Dr Malinga is still there 3 years later. He has outlasted most African health ministers, whose average term of office is only 18 months. During that time he and his team have had to provide services across a large country where rebels are still active in the north, there have been outbreaks of Ebola fever and torrential rain has caused flooding and widespread damage.

These two stories, one about an NGO and one about an African Government, describe people taking action to deal with the problems they see. They are, of course, remarkable people, but in my experience there are remarkably many others like them or who want to be like them around the world.

The last chapter set out a new vision of global health that was based on values associated with our interdependence, our desire for independence and the rights and responsibilities we all share. Here we look at what this might mean in practice and how the ideas in this book might actually make a difference in the real world.

Most of the best ideas we have come across in *Turning the World Upside Down* are intensely practical. They are what people have learned from doing things.

Fazle Hassan Abed of BRAC and Arvind Ohja of URVAL are leaders who have had a clear vision about what is needed and experimented with different approaches until they found the right answer. Amongst the clinicians and scientists, Don Berwick of the Institute for Healthcare Improvement (IHI) and Lee Hartwell of the Partnership for Personalized Medicine have developed their ideas from observing what works in practice. Amongst politicians Ministers Tedros of Ethiopia and Garrido of Mozambique have used what they have to hand to make as much progress as they can.

As a former Chief Executive I naturally admire the practical people who get things done and, as a former servant of Government, I am reminded of the standard politician's question: "That's a good idea, but how do we implement it, how do we put it into practice, how do we make sure it happens?"

One of the Secretaries of State with whom I worked in the NHS, John Reid, was fond of quoting Gramsci's aphorism that the optimism of the will needs to be matched by the pessimism of the intellect. He told me that politicians had plenty of the will and determination. They had the ability to have visions and build castles in the air and change the political climate, but they needed other people, and by implication me and my colleagues, to be aware of the problems, to be pessimistic and to find the practical ways to make things happen.

I have described this book as a search to understand what is happening in health. One thing that is very clear as we come to the end of our search is that change is happening. Old ideas about the role of professionals and the neutrality of science have been changing for 20 years or more. Even doctors don't believe that it's enough to say "Trust me, I'm a doctor" any more and scientists are well aware that their pure scientific discovery can be used for good purposes or for bad. We are all subject to scrutiny and to question.

Much more recently we have lost our unquestioning faith that the 'invisible hand' of the market will always find the right answer, which has been such a totem of the right for the last 30 years. At the same time, however, economic reality is making us face up to the fact that more spending, and particularly more government spending – that totem of the left – is neither possible nor necessarily desirable. Capitalism may be being tamed, but so, too, is big government.

We are clear that we are not living in the past anymore; but we haven't yet started to live in the future. We are, in the language I have used in this book, stuck between paradigms. One model doesn't fit anymore, but the new one isn't available yet.

The direction of travel is pretty straightforward and I know many intelligent and wise people, some of whom are quoted in this book, who can design for us the model for the future. We are travelling in a direction that will take us from a top-down world where doctor, scientist, business leader, government always knows best, to one where we will judge things much more for ourselves, share ideas and perceptions freely with our peers and expect some basic human rights to be observed.

We are travelling in the direction shown in Figure 10.1 from the top-down world of western scientific medicine to the more egalitarian one of global health. The trouble is that it will not be as smooth a transition as the figure suggest, a gentle glide into a new world. We know that there are many interests that are opposing the transition. We also know that the change will be disruptive and difficult. If we are to move from a physician and hospital centric model, as many people have been trying to do for 30 or more years in richer countries and in poorer ones, we will meet resistance.

Leaving aside the obvious vested interests, it is likely to mean turning down long nurtured local plans for expansion, perhaps shutting local hospitals and taking away some entitlements whilst replacing them with others. Many members of the public won't be on side.

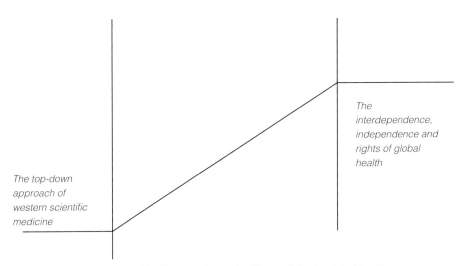

Figure 10.1 The ideal transition from western scientific medicine to global health

Nevertheless, change is happening. There are powerful forces opposing change, but there are now powerful forces driving it. Patients, young professionals, payers and politicians are now moving in a similar direction. The scene is set for conflict. These latter forces will, no doubt, ultimately win, if for no other reason than that we can't afford the current model. However, in the meantime the path to change will look much more like that described in Figure 10.2, a chequered progress of gains and losses before the ultimate victory.

The big questions for us now are how to accelerate the change, smooth its path and make sure that not too much damage is done on the way? Part of the answer, at least, is to do what the pioneers always do. We, too, need to learn by doing.

In this final chapter I summarise some of the key findings from earlier chapters that I believe will help us make this transition as fast and as comfortably as possible. I conclude

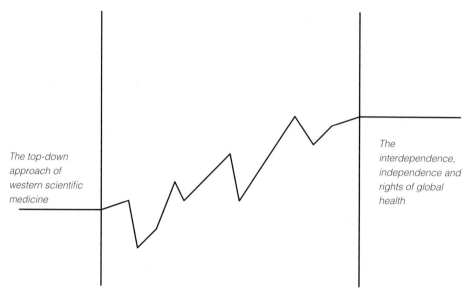

The top-down approach of western scientific medicine

The interdependence, independence and rights of global health

Figure 10.2 The real-life transition from western scientific medicine to global health

by proposing three actions that will involve thousands of people discovering the future for themselves as they help to create it.

Where do we go from here?

Our exploration has led us to a few very high level conclusions and a number of more specific observations that appear to be crucial for the future.

First of all, there is the point that, whether a country is rich or poor, health sits within a much wider social, economic and political context and affects and is affected by whatever else is happening in education, broader society, politics, the physical environment and the economy. The use of tobacco, the deaths of so many women in childbirth or when pregnant and the health effects of climate change are all obvious examples of this; but, we also know that heart disease and mental health are related to social and economic factors.

Within this context we can see that efforts to improve health will have to operate at three levels simultaneously: dealing directly with health issues; promoting wealth and countering poverty and its effects; and supporting beneficial social change. One without the others will have limited effect. Together they reinforce each other.

The second broad point is that we are facing an epidemic of non-communicable disease, which our systems generally are not designed or capable of dealing with well. Moreover, as we have observed, different patients need different services. One size doesn't fit all.

However, as we have also seen, the very powerful health services of richer countries have now become part of the problem, getting in the way of necessary change. There, paradoxically, health systems are too strong and too greedy – forcing physicians and patients into inappropriate and expensive activities – and, too often, devaluing the real skills of the one and ignoring the real needs of the other.

The final overarching point is that our vision for what we are trying to achieve in health needs to be constructed around the idea of independence and of supporting people – the disabled, the dying, the fit, fat or just average – to be able to live their lives as independently as possible and, as far as possible, in the way they want. This is profoundly important, because, by moving away from a more usual or more clinical description, it will influence the sort of services that need to be provided.

This independence is reflected in the fact that the patient is at the centre of what happens, not because clinicians or politicians put them there, but because for most of the time they will actually determine what really happens, based on their own perception and the trade-offs they make. They are also the judges of their own standard of life, as we are reminded by Baroness Campbell's story of overhearing a doctor say her quality of life was so poor that they wouldn't try to save her.

Against the background of these three conclusions there are five much more specific observations about what is needed in the new world. Each of these is a part of the solution, each links with each other and each will help accelerate change.

The first observation is about the power of the quality improvement methodologies used by the IHI and others to bring about local clinically driven change and to spread better practice around a community. Designing better services and systems can sometimes seem to be just about mobilising resources, training people and getting the pieces in place and setting up processes and systems. These improvement methodologies go much further than this. They engage the people running the services in their design and, crucially, in constantly improving the service by bringing in new ideas and testing out what works in practice.

I have put this point at the top of the list because it is so often overlooked in practice or seen as an add on. It is central. I am not alone in worrying that donors will pour money into poorer countries, building up their infrastructure and staffing, but not make the most of the opportunity to re-design the service and make sure that it is capable of constantly re-designing itself.

These poorer countries will be designing and building their services as they train and recruit their health workers. There could not be a better time to build in the knowledge and practice of continuous improvement than now. As Francis Omaswa says "poor people can't afford waste". None of us can.

The second observation is also about people. It is the point that comes through so clearly from any time spent with health workers in poorer countries. We should train and deploy people to do the task in hand and not purely for the professions. In many countries around the world, *tecnicos di cirurgia*, clinical officers, cataract surgeons and others – if well trained, motivated and able to refer their patients on where necessary – are successfully carrying a large part of the burden of healthcare. In richer countries, with our minds conditioned by our history, we automatically view the world in terms of the traditional professions and allow their language of 'task shifting' and 'professional standards' to dominate and shape our thinking.

This is not an argument against cultivating the highest standards, the greatest expertise and the greatest professionalism. It is an argument against training thousands and, indeed, millions of doctors for lengthy periods and then expecting them to work far below their skill levels on things that others could do with far less training. This is changing in richer countries and it is particularly interesting to see that when doctors control budgets, as GP practices now do in England, they are much bolder about letting lower skilled staff, who cost less, take on more tasks.

The central point here, however, is to create a health system based on the idea of training and deploying health workers to do the tasks needed – there will be need for the most skilled as well as others – rather than one based on professions, with aides and helpers filling in at the margins.

The third area is science and technology, with all the potential and actual benefits it brings. Here, as we saw earlier, the key questions in health are how it can be used and whether, in particular, it helps promote early health or only deals with late disease; whether it encourages the independence we want or only leads to greater dependency on experts and commercial solutions; and whether it creates more equity in the world or only further widens inequalities.

These important questions can be overlooked in the rush to build bigger and better health systems and invent new technologies. They can, alternatively, be built into health system design as the Partnership for Personalized Medicine is seeking to do.

The fourth observation is about the importance of bringing clinical medicine and public health much closer together. Once again, experience in poorer countries shows us how this can be done at the most local level by breaking down – or never having erected – barriers between different groups of staff. This also happens to some extent in richer countries, but once again it is not generally systematic or system wide.

Finally, and underpinning all the rest, is the importance of creating viable business models to ensure that developments are viable in the longer term. This may seem obvious, but, as uncontrolled expenditure growth in many richer countries shows, it has very often not happened in practice.

One of the major problems, as we have seen, is that the forces of professional advancement, scientific and technological development and commerce combine to promote ever-growing expenditure, regardless of its value. A viable business model depends very much on its environment – what works in one place may not work in another – and there will be different solutions achieved in different countries. Processes like Triple Aim, where a group of organisations work together to explore how to bring together population health, individual healthcare and cost control are invaluable for the rest of us in exploring what may be possible in the future.

Each of these observations is important it itself, but each will also accelerate and smooth the transition path.

I have drawn out these particular observations and insights because they are important and because most of them are not things that are generally yet given enough attention in my view in the discussions about re-designing and strengthening health systems in rich or poor countries. This needs to change.

Three proposals for action

As we move towards proposing action there is something that is so simple that it almost doesn't need to be said. Global health is about all of us. We need to stop having compartmentalised discussions about health in poor countries over here and health in richer ones over there. In health almost everything is linked or shared.

This relates to the other obvious point, which is now very well understood – that health is about teamwork and the bringing together of different perspectives and skills to a common purpose. We should think about countries in a similar way as having parts to play, insights to offer and resources to share.

I have used a metaphor of unfair trade throughout *Turning the World Upside Down*, pointing out that poor countries export health workers and richer ones export ideas and ideologies. I have suggested that it should be turned the other way round so that richer countries export a part of their great wealth of health workers and poorer ones export ideas that they have learned from their experience in a much harder environment for the delivery of healthcare.

I still think that turning the trade upside down in this way would be a good idea, but I know that this is only a step towards a new, more equal and more complex relationship. I also know that the world is changing fast economically and politically and could, if we choose to make it do so, support this change. The alternative, of course, is that we may see a new set of partitions and divides created that will slow this process of coming together and do enormous damage in health and elsewhere.

The stakes are high in geo-political terms, but, returning to the world of health, it is interesting to note that whilst politicians and world health leaders are working hard to create greater alignment, there is what I have called a movement of people and ideas developing at a much more local level. Interconnections, communication and contact are growing at the speed of the Internet, the cell phone and the aeroplane. Partnerships, migration and voluntary activity are all increasing.

This is not yet fully visible. The caricature is that health globally is about politicians and pop stars parading on the world stage, with the professional lobbyists and campaigners trying to control and influence from the sidelines. It is about Brown, Obama, the World Health Organization, the World Bank, Oxfam, One Campaign and others, who between them have been very successful in keeping these issues near the top of the world agenda, mobilising resources and coordinating action. Where, however, are the practitioners, the people who are doing things locally?

They may not yet be visible, but their role is invaluable not just in what they do but in bringing greater understanding across countries and continents. In the UK, Build is a network of organisations, including health ones that are involved in some way in partnering and linking people in different communities. Its goal is to make these partnerships mainstream in our life and in our thinking.[1]

Build quotes one of its members, Jo Sang from Kenya, as saying:

> "The attitude towards Africa must change. It is a continent with problems, yes, but also with incredible spirit in the face of difficulties. The humanity, the love, the warmth, the laughter, the celebration of life, the hard work, the intelligence, the determination to move is all there. What is needed is not charity. If one goes into development work thinking 'Aid', one nurtures the very situation that keeps dependency alive. Sustained intercultural community partnerships can bring the needed change in attitude to make this shift from aid/charity to development on a more equal and dignified basis." [2]

A movement of people and ideas

There is, as I said in the last chapter, a movement of people and ideas converging around the same group of themes and issues.

My first proposal, which builds on these ideas, is that we need to turn this movement into a Movement. There are many groups already active in the field but not, I think, with quite this emphasis on creating a new way of thinking about and working in health in ways that are the same in richer or in poorer countries. Such a movement would take as its starting point the three sets of values associated with interdependence, independence and the right to health. It would be about quality and equality and it would seek to engage practitioners of every sort, from the clinician to the hospital engineer who knows about clean water supplies, in sharing their ideas and practice and in creating the future.

I am familiar with a number of organisations that have overlapping aims and where people meet regardless of their background, discipline and speciality to share and create. I believe that now is the time to bring these together in an alliance of alliances to add weight to their individual efforts. Now is the right time for groups like the Global Health Council, IHI and hundreds of small networks to find a way of working together and ensure that global health is about the practitioners at the local level as well as about the politicians, policymakers and campaigners. This is happening in other sectors where Linux or social networking, *Make Poverty History* and other campaigns are attracting mass involvement. In health, pioneers like IHI have developed *Futureworks* to find 'crowd sourcing' solutions to problems. The time is right to take this further.

Perhaps more controversially, there is a role here, too, for the big commercial leaders – who, and it has long struck me as curious, don't behave as if they were health leaders – and for the professional bodies to adopt new approaches, recognising that the world is changing and that their very future will depend on creating new relationships in a changing landscape.

A coming together, in whatever way is possible, by some of these groups could have profound impact, help accelerate the change and make sure that the next few years look more like the trajectory in Figure 10.1 than that in Figure 10.2.

Re-designing the education and training of health workers

The second proposal is to re-design the education and training of health workers in order to change the way they think about the world and equip them with the skills they need for the twenty-first century.

It was 100 years ago that Abraham Flexner, with the backing of the Carnegie Foundation, took American medical education apart. He visited every one of the 150 establishments in the USA that taught medicine and reviewed their quality and capability, identifying those that taught medicine scientifically and those that based their curricula on a mix of received wisdom, enlightened experience and sheer quackery.

His explosive report of 1910 led to the closure of around one-third of the existing medical schools. It established the tenets of teaching medicine in the USA that last to this day. These tenets are based on the understanding that medicine is a science, subject like every other natural science to rules of scientific inquiry, the testing of hypotheses and evidence collection.

Now 100 years later many people have been changing and developing the curricula used in professional education. It has changed enormously since 30 years ago, when doctors of my age tell me that they memorised the names of every bone in he foot but learned nothing about nutrition and certainly didn't have programmes about 'breaking bad news', communications, ethics and gender.

The common thread is about how medicine is adapting to the norms of a new world and about placing medicine in context. It is also about learning the skills that employers actually want – the ability to operate in the real world as a competent practitioner able to improve services as well as deliver them. The dominance now of diseases, which I have described earlier as being parasitic on our behaviour and on society, rather than just on our physical body and physical environment, is accelerating the need for change.

I propose that we now need a full and authoritative re-design of the education and training of health workers to match that undertaken by Flexner a century ago. Today such a review would need to bring in the ideas and experience of China, Asia, Africa and Latin and South America as well as of Europe and North America.

There have been incremental changes over the last few years; a full-scale review might now prove to be as profound as Flexner's was. It would, in the sense of the paradigm shift we have been discussing, be about putting medicine and science fully in its context, where it is empowered by its patients and rendered effective by society.

Julio Frenk, the Head of the Harvard School of Public Health and formerly the inspirational Minister of Health in Mexico, who developed conditional cash transfers and much else, has established a working group to initiate the project. It needs the support of the global health authorities and the involvement of global health workers.

Creating African, Asian and American alliances to train and educate more health workers where they are needed

One of the luxuries of the author is to advocate actions for other people to implement. I understand this only too well as the former Chief Executive of the NHS who received numbers of proposals, recommendations and reports every week for more than 5 years. I remember that in one year alone, I received more than 200 recommendations from the Audit Commission. We have all received unsolicited advice. Some is good and some is complete nonsense. The latter, of course, takes up as much time as the former.

In keeping with the spirit of this book I have already taken a small step in implementing my third proposal and will do more.

There is a well-documented shortfall in trained health workers globally with, as we have seen earlier, the biggest problems in the poorest countries. The WHO has estimated that there is a shortage of at least of 4.3 million health workers.

There are, as we have discussed, many issues to do with the distribution and employment of health workers throughout the world and particular problems caused by the migration of trained health workers from poor to rich countries. Underlying all these problems however is a failure to train sufficient numbers in most countries of the world.

There is also an extraordinary tradition in the UK and other rich countries of health workers volunteering to work in poor countries and of health institutions linking with others in poorer countries to help provide support and development. There are now literally hundreds of examples from Canada, the USA, Holland, Germany, and Scandinavian countries; French institutions link with others in French-speaking countries and Portuguese-speaking countries link together.

I described briefly in Chapter 6 the role that THET, MEMISA and ESTHER had in the UK, Belgium and France, respectively, in coordinating and supporting these initiatives. They have been very active in training health workers in their partners' own countries. To take one example, THET has supported London's Kings College Hospital to link with the Government of Somalia and, with the help of UNICEF, has helped to educate and graduate the first medical students in the country for 20 years.

Why can't we put the need and the willingness to help together? There seems to be an obvious match. Foreign health workers could help train an enormous increase in health workers in countries where they are needed in a relatively short time. There would not need to be a long-term building up of trainers and, when the bulk of the training was done, the training capacity could be scaled down to the appropriate level needed for the long term. There is a bulge of training to deal with as illustrated in Figure 10.3.

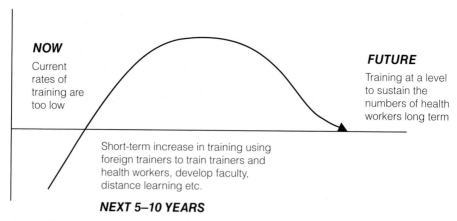

Figure 10.3 Training can be increased rapidly in the short term whilst Africa builds capacity

By the summer of 2008 I had become convinced that there was much more that could be done to use all this goodwill and expertise in rich countries to help address the need for education and training in poor ones. I decided to test out my ideas with other people. I therefore sent out a short note with a very simple questionnaire to about 35 UK health and education leaders whom I knew personally and asked for a quick reply.

It really was a very simple questionnaire and asked only three questions. Given the need for educating and training many more health workers in Africa, should the UK be doing more to help in Africa? If so, what should we be doing? Finally, are you already doing something about this or are you planning to do something in the future? I asked for the replies on two sides of A4 paper.

I also wrote to 12 African leaders, some ministers, some permanent secretaries and some heads of medical and nursing schools and asked them the same questions in the course of a personal email.

The results were compelling. All the African and British people said that more could be done, and most said more should be done. They produced the same list of what this might be, ranging from training the trainers, to providing adjunct faculty to teach in existing schools, support for curriculum development and distance learning. Two-thirds of the British respondents said that they were already doing something and two-thirds said they planned to do more.

The most remarkable fact was that I sent out 35 emails to UK people on 3 August and got 133 responses by the end of the month. People had passed it on down their networks and there was enough enthusiasm to move people to reply in this month of holidays. Equally importantly, more than one-third of respondents were the principals of their organisations: deans of schools, chief executives of hospitals and presidents of universities.

This was an overwhelming response and I needed to do something. Taking advice from some of the respondents I decided to try to set up a scheme in one country to test the concept. Dr Simon Miti, the Permanent Secretary in Zambia had been one of the respondents and was keen to work up a scheme. Together with the Zambian High Commissioner to the UK, the Honourable Anderson Chibwa, and my colleagues Dr David Percy and Ms Susana Edjang, we created the Zambia UK Health Workforce Alliance with the purposes described in Figure 10.4.

As I write, the scheme has been funded and the first health workers will be going to Zambia next year. The Zambian Government is very supportive and the UK's NHS and Department for International Development have been very helpful.

About 40 organisations are involved in the Alliance and have committed themselves to sharing information and working together. Over time I hope that all Zambian and UK organisations working together will participate and help make what might otherwise be small contributions into something with a long-term and strategic impact.

The Alliance will bring together health workers, health and education institutions, NGOs and private sector organisations in Zambia and the UK to:

- *support Zambia to implement its Health Human Resources Strategy and contribute to achieving the health-related Millennium Development Goals*

- *provide opportunities for learning and development for health workers and institutions in both Zambia and the UK*

- *test the concept of such an Alliance between health systems for application elsewhere*

Figure 10.4 The Zambia UK Health Workforce Alliance

This scheme may not look very different to others, where training has been going on for years; the main differences are threefold: the focus is entirely on pre-service education and training, getting more people into the workforce; it is coordinated and, it is mutual with the NHS and its staff expected to gain from the relationship.

It is too early to tell how successful the Zambia UK Alliance will be. There are real and practical difficulties to work through about terms and conditions, about working in another country and about re-entry into your own. There is a lot of devil in the detail. It is not as easy as it may sound. There is no doubt, however, that there is increasing impetus from organisations around the world to link in this way and increasing interest amongst health workers to experience other systems and countries and to explore what global health means in reality. We in rich countries, as I have shown in earlier chapters, have a great deal to learn from working with our counterparts in poor ones.

Since we created the Alliance I have had five other countries come to me and ask me to set up similar schemes. We need to be cautious and to make sure that we learn how to do this effectively as we go along. We also need to make sure that we build in improvement and don't just create health workers suitable to work in richer countries and not able to lead their countries in their own development. They need health workers trained for the job that needs to be done and not just for the professions.

We also need to be sure that there will be health services to work in and jobs for the people once they are trained. By working within the national plan, this sort of approach will fit into the wider picture, where the Government and its partners must balance all aspects of their health system development. There is an opportunity here. The development partners globally have recognised the need to scale up health worker training and committed funds for health system expansion. We could expand this massively and quickly, creating alliances involving health workers from many different countries in training in Africa, Asia or South America, wherever it is needed and seen as a priority.

Richer countries could use their skills, learn for themselves and, of course, pay back a debt for the thousands of workers who have come to their countries to work. Moreover it will engage thousands of people and help build the new global health understanding that we need. This is a win–win situation. We should make the most of it.

Action

These three actions are all perfectly practical. They are happening in smaller and less coordinated ways already.

There is already a movement, which needs to become a Movement.

There is enormous interest in re-designing professional education to equip health workers to meet the demands of the twenty-first century. Someone somewhere needs to seize the opportunity and find the way to channel all the insight and creativity into producing a new and clear model or framework for the future. It will equip health workers to deliver improved global health.

Finally, thousands of individuals are turning the world upside down for themselves by learning from poor countries and innovators wherever they are in the world. They are gaining experience that will be invaluable for them wherever they work and enable them truly to be a new breed of global health professionals.

These three actions will deliver change, add impetus to what is already happening and help us to move more smoothly up the slope from seeing the world in terms of twentieth-century western scientific medicine to realising fully our approach to global health. They are all about making change where it really matters – in the minds and behaviours of health workers and the public.

References

1. www.build-online.org.uk.
2. Build. Leaflet. May 2008.

INDEX

About the Author

Lord Nigel Crisp has unique experience of health in both rich and poor countries. He ran England's National Health Service for more than 5 years and was, exceptionally, head of the UK Department of Health at the same time. The NHS is the world's biggest health system and the fourth biggest organisation in the world with 1.3 million staff and £90 billion annual turnover.

He has subsequently worked extensively in poor countries as an advisor to Tony Blair and consultant to the World Health Organization and the Gates Foundation. He is currently supporting Sarah Brown with the Maternal Mortality Campaign and has founded the Zambia UK Health Workforce Alliance to promote mutual learning and development.

He has published two very influential reports - *Global Health Partnerships* in 2007 and *Scaling up, Saving Lives* in 2008 as well as several chapters and articles in journals such as The BMJ and The Lancet and is in demand globally as a thinker and speaker on global health.

Nigel Crisp is an independent Peer in the House of Lords, Chair of Sightsavers International, a Professor at the London School of Hygiene and Tropical Medicine, a Senior Fellow of the Institute for Healthcare Improvement in Cambridge, Massachusetts, Consultant to HLM Architects and an Honorary Fellow of St John's College, Cambridge and of the Royal College of Physicians.

More information is available at http://www.nigelcrisp.com

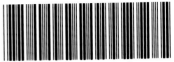

Turning the World Upside Down:
the search for global health in the twenty-first century

DATE DUE

Sept 2012			
26/8/17			
18/1/22			

Demco, Inc. 38-293